Unveiled Truth

What doctors don't know will hurt you!

Nina L. Venturella

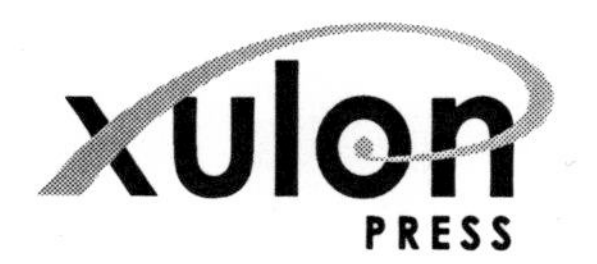

Unveiled Truth
What doctors don't know will hurt you!
by Nina L. Venturella

Printed in the United States of America

ISBN 9781625091314

www.xulonpress.com

Contents

INTRODUCTION

After many years of struggling with my own health, I now have victory and insight and the capability to share my story with others. My passion and desire to change lives has driven me to write this book, Unveiled Truth, what doctors don't know will hurt you! Unveils hidden truths of how the body can be healed and cleansed in ways traditional medicine could not.

I am not a doctor, and I don't have a PhD. I am, however, a Certified Personal Trainer, Certified Nutritionist, and the founder and developer of X'Tract, a cleansing technique for the lymphatic system that has proven results and success.

Over the 23 years of working with clients that have established proven success stories of struggles and accomplishments in achieving optimal health, I discovered how important and crucial it is to cleanse in unison the body, soul, and spirit. The soul consists of the mind, the will, and the emotions.

By cleansing these three parts of your being, the reality for living a long healthy prosperous life is more than possible. Once success is established within these three main areas, "Trinity for Health" is the end result.

Let's embark on this seven-week journey together and discover the revealed truths.

How to benefit most from this book

This book is divided into 2 main parts. (Toxic Holding Tanks) Body Tank and the Soul Tank. (There are toxins in our physical body as well as our soul).

I have categorized each of the root causes according to each of the specific tanks. I have included action items, thoughts to ponder, scriptures, and next steps at the end of each chapter.

I strongly recommend that you read and do each action item necessary for cleansing each of the tanks separately. I have designed this book not only to educate you on these 2 toxic tanks, but also to help you go thru the process of elimination and discovering each of the 14 root causes in order to achieve your own Trinity for health. This is a diagnostic tool for you to use over and over again I have given an in depth checklist for health, called *Process of elimination.*

In order to get the maximum results be sure to interact with the book and let it become a daily regimen and transformation in your mind, body and soul.

The following are the main points that will assist in your success in achieving optimal health and going through the journey of cleansing and the getting to the root cause verses treating symptoms. The four main points are:

- **Establishing and understanding specific root causes**- this is the gold nugget that creates awareness and gives a task oriented check list for the process of elimination.
- **Self-Discovery**- these questions will help you determine if you have one of the root causes and if so, how to cleanse and eliminate it.
- **Scriptures to speak over yourself**- Words, positive affirmations, and bible verses that will improve your health and life and start you on your prosperous journey.
- **Next steps**- Action items and goals to achieve daily.

I pray that this book will deliver you in such a way that you will never again say why. You will be delivered and set free as it is Gods will for all his children to live in freedom and no longer in captivity. Gods will for all his children is for us to live a long healthy prosperous life and for our soul and body to be whole and toxic free.

"Beloved *I wish above all things that you prosper and be in health even as thy soul does prosper."- 3rd* John 2:1

My strongest desire is that as you read this book and you would experience a peace that is so deep inside you that you can't help but smile. You get a renewed strength in your heart and a new found hope comes into you.

Experiencing total freedom in your body and soul, having and achieving prosperity in all areas, that is what we were called to do, and that is what this book is designed to do.

Be sure to do all the action items at the end of each chapter, Read all the scriptures and words of affirmation, and stick with it until you see all the benefits you are seeking.

So let's embark together on this journey for cleansing the soul and body in a way that can only result in optimal health and well-being, for total wholeness, vitality and longevity.

My Personal Journey

Many experts say you are not an expert until you have walked in the shoes I have walked in. Books are written with revelations about health and well-being, because people have had their own health struggles; in trying to find out what is wrong with them, they have stumbled into a way to help others. I believe that is exactly how my story began. In my early twenties, I was certified as a personal trainer and nutritionist. I had extensive knowledge in nutrition from classes and seminars I attended regularly. My issue was not eating the wrong foods, or having a bad lifestyle—mine was an issue that is plaguing thousands of people today.

I learned very quickly that health is very dependent on the types of foods you eat and how often—or little—waste is eliminated. I also realized my words and thoughts had a lot to do with how good or bad I felt on a particular day. My situation was a gradual process; it began with becoming allergic and having reactions to most foods I ate. I noticed I was extremely fatigued and had a lowered immune system, almost as if it was shutting down. The real clincher for me was the incredibly agonizing constipated feeling that would never stop. I was down to eliminating less than one time every two to three weeks. The first sign of disease is in your skin; since it is your largest organ, it is the "tell all" of health. That was when I really knew something was very wrong with me and that I needed to get help, as I was breaking out with acne all over.

Frustrated, I started my journey, researching doctors and medical specialists for allergies, the immune system, and for general medical advice. After pursuing information and having many unfruitful visits, I was simply being told I was stressed out or tired. One doctor even told me that my body will eliminate on its own time and that I had nothing to worry about. Feeling very hopeless and discouraged with all my medical efforts, I started thinking maybe it was just stress or all in my head. The one gift I know I have is that I'm very intuitive with my own health and the health of others. I knew instantly that something was off and not in balance. I was sick and tired of being sick and tired. This went on for years; the symptoms were progressing and were becoming more acute. I knew I had to do something, but what? I had gone the medical route and was not aware or educated on other alternatives, yet.

The doctors had agreed that exercise was good for me. One day while working out, someone told me about a naturopathic doctor. Of course I had no idea who or what that was. I was told that a naturopathic doctor is one who is not traditional but uses alternative natural methods of diagnosis and treatment. My initial thought was if anyone was opposite of medical doctors, sign me up. Don't get me wrong: doctors are good for many things; they just didn't help me.

On the way over to see the naturopathic doctor, my mind kept playing tricks on me. I was trying to self-diagnose. I was going over any medical history issues I may have had in my family, in past generations. I was thinking of something I may have contracted from someone in my past. Every time you go to a new doctor they always ask about your family history and past surgeries or traumas that may have had adverse effects on your body or condition. After racking my brain for over an hour and coming up blank, I finally arrived at my destination and the beginning of my "awakening. "

As I walked up the steps to her door, I saw the words Homeopathic MD. I also saw the words Iridology and muscle testing. My first thought was, *Oh yay; she is a freak; she is probably going to do some voodoo thing on me.* For a brief moment I actually thought of leaving and turn back. As I was contemplating going back home, the door opened, and a very young, pretty girl came out and asked if she could help me. I hesitantly said, "Yes, I have an appointment with someone here; is that you?" She smiled, and we went inside. I saw tons of herbs, root teas, and modalities I had never seen before. I told her my symptoms and within minutes she looked in my eyes and at my tongue and told me I had Candida. I had panic in my voice, thinking it was some incurable fatal disease, and said, "What the heck is that?" Again she smiled, so I knew it couldn't be that bad. After all, no one gives bad news with a smile. She told me it is yeast throughout the body. I instantly thought she was crazy, and I thought I had never had a yeast infection in my life. She said it is not vaginal; it is in your gut. In short, she said, "It is an overgrowth of bad bacteria overtaking the good."She gave me a stack of papers with a grocery list with about five items on it and probiotics. She told me that should do it.

I was driving home skeptical but optimistic. I thought that maybe she knew what she was talking about because she was very confident in all her answers. To my great surprise she was right on. As soon as I began the diet and taking the probiotics I started feeling better within just a week.

I began thinking a lot about the health and well-being of others. If I had this yeast in my body causing all these issues, then how many more people are out there like me with the same or even worse symptoms? It turns out I got all this yeast as a side effect from tetracycline and also found out most meds and antibiotics release yeast, which causes Candida. I began learning that Candida comes in various levels and degrees, from mild to advanced levels. Its symptoms were far more severe and seemed to be endless with the more advances cases.

This was the beginning of an obsessive desire to help others with their health and well-being; helping them obtain optimal health and setting them free from Candida, once and for all. Back then I was taught that once you have Candida, you can be susceptible to getting it again Thank the Lord that my eyes have been opened and now see the truth that has been unveiled. I am now going to share with you the key to unlocking and ridding the body of Candida for good. Keep reading!

You know the saying, "Everything happens for a reason. " Because of the pursuit to overcome my own health challenges, I have successfully helped hundreds upon hundreds of people with the same or similar conditions and issues.

There was even greater light at the end of the tunnel. It made me really think about life in a different way, realizing I am not immortal, and health is really a major key in life. I no longer take health or life for granted. It truly made me seek my faith and surrender to God wholeheartedly.

I began to pay attention to my words and thoughts about my own health, and it became very obvious how negative I had been speaking without even realizing it. I was creating my own destiny with the words that were coming out of my mouth. Sickness was what I was declaring for my own body. It was a startling revelation.

I had been saved a very short time prior to getting sick and turned to God for help with what was happening to me. While pursuing my walk with God, I have come to realize that we live in a spiritual world with forces all around. My long, long journey began with understanding the spiritual world and all it entails and how our spiritual lives can affect physical health and well-being.

In remission from Candida, many years later, I was introduced to a lady from Europe who hired me to do sales and marketing for her wellness beauty clinic, which catered to the very wealthy and vain. While there, I learned of a system I had never heard about—the lymphatic system—and I was extremely fascinated.

What I learned in a very short time was that this system is crucial for the many major organs in the body. The importance of the lymphatic system is very much underestimated in the medical world and in the United States. This was the missing link to healing the whole body and staying healthy without the yo-yo effect of recurring illness.

In the later chapters you will learn more about the lymphatic system and why it is vitally crucial to the entire body.

Soon after my return from Europe, my research into the lymphatic system and all its benefits was my focus, and it has been for the last 14 years. Treating people with this technique and teaching people has been my life's purpose. It came as a great surprise, and I had no idea how my life had been impacted and how others would benefit from my discovering this system. Many people have asked me how I know so much about the lymphatic system and how it works. I can tell you this: I get my wisdom from God, not books, and He has taught me and gifted me to develop a technique that cleanses the body's entire lymphatic system.

My journey to healing and health led me to open a Wellness Center in 2006. All my research and personal testimonies began coming together. I would finally use the experience and research for a greater purpose. Life is a great big jigsaw puzzle with pieces everywhere, and it has the capacity to form many pictures, but there is only one "right" picture. My whole life I had been forming wrong pictures until 2006 when the picture began to take the "right" form. I had a dream that was very real and very descriptive when I was just a teenager; it was about starting my own Wellness Center, which has come to pass!

Earlier you heard me say that sin started sickness. I also believe that it can end there. Healing in the soul (mind, will, and emotions) is as important, if not more so, than physical healing. It is mandatory and necessary that they all are examined and cleansed for optimal health, the "Trinity for Health. "

The Importance of Cleansing

Medical professionals, both traditional and alternative, say how important food is to the body. There is virtually every type of supplement available on the market today with various brands and recommendations. You are what you eat, and, generally, supplements are good. However, I personally do not take vitamins, and I take very few supplements. You will see in later chapters my personal favorites.

In order to have true health in the body and soul, elimination of toxic waste in the physical body is a must. But it doesn't stop there. Elimination of toxic waste in the soul (negative thoughts, hurts from words, and wounds from traumas, etc.) is essential. Prior to allowing anything good to enter in (such as healthy foods, supplements, positive thoughts and words), you must first eliminate the bad.

The body is designed to digest and eliminate. If the body, specifically the colon, does not release waste daily, the body's main function is to store for survival, until the digestive cycle takes place again. This process is outlined in later chapters.

The body can be so full of toxins that it cannot possibly process foods and assimilate the necessary vitamins and nutrients. The result is that urine does not eliminate toxins, and vital nutrients do not get into the body. Too many toxins are coming in, and not enough are going out!

If the mind does not get cleansed from negative thoughts, words, and memories, then sickness is the result. A toxic mind (negative thoughts and words) will manifest sickness and disease in the physical body.

The overwhelming toxicity in the body and soul (mind, will, and emotions) will stop you from moving forward in life and stop you from experiencing the abundant life that's available for you.

Understanding how it all began is the first step to the journey of removing toxicity and achieving the "Trinity for Health."

When Sickness Began

Venture back to the Garden of Eden in Genesis when Adam and Eve disobeyed God. Instantly sickness and disease began, and the knowledge of death became a reality. Prior to that act, sickness was not even a thought, nor was there any understanding of such a thing as death.

The events as they happened in the Bible:

- The knowledge of the world was already established in the Kingdom.
- God spoke the world into existence.
- God made Adam.
- God made a companion for Adam and called her Eve.
- God gave them all the freedom to eat of any tree in the garden but not of the tree of the knowledge of good and evil.
- Satan tempted Eve.
- Eve gave in to temptation.
- Obedience and sin began.

- Man became cursed.
- Sickness and death became real.

Life has never been the same since that time. Understanding how it all began is the key to the foundation of healing. This is an interactive how-to book written just for you.

This book is divided into three main parts or what can be called Toxic Holding Tanks. They are the body, the soul, and the spirit. In addition, there are 14 root causes of sickness and disease in each of these tanks.

Each of the root causes are categorized according to each of the specific tanks. I have included action items, thoughts to ponder, scriptures, and the next steps at the end of each chapter.

To use this book properly as a tool for healing, read and do each action item necessary for cleansing each of the tanks separately. This book is designed to shed light on these three toxic tanks, and each of the fourteen root causes. This will provide the necessary tools for healing and optimum health.

Process of Elimination

DIAGNOSTIC CHECKLIST—14 ROOT CAUSES OF SICKNESS AND DISEASE

If a body is toxic, it doesn't have a fighting chance to live an abundant, quality life. Newsflash: if you struggle and go to a doctor for a magic pill for energy, weight loss, better sleep, and so on, you are not riding the body of the problem, but adding toxins to it! Ponder this for a moment: 60 percent of people who are in the hospital are in because of side effects due to prescription drugs given by a doctor or specialist.

Ask yourself this question: "Do I want a doctor to continue to give me drugs with known side effects that are most likely worse than the current condition I am using them for."

If your answer is "Yes," this book is definitely not for you. Put it down, walk away, or give it away to someone who is ready for the truth.

If you answered "No," then this is the key that will answer the vexing question, "What the heck is wrong with me?" Your solution is in this book. Your answers to years of questions are here. The good news is that your struggles can be over.

The Process of Elimination can be simple and pain free:

- The root cause checklist
- The self-diagnosis
- The appropriate recommendations

This is the "Trinity of Health. " All three "tanks" must be cleansed and free for complete and total health and prosperity. Most diseases begin in the soul, with negative words spoken to us by ourselves or spoken by others. They are followed by a reaction, symptom, or sickness. It is necessary that the physical and the soul tanks be cleansed simultaneously so that the body can have a brand new beginning.

I invite you to sit back, relax, and take all this in as we journey together to a new way of life and establish total and complete health in all areas. Fasten your seatbelts; it's going to be an eye-opening adventure you will not want to miss!

RELEASE, RENEW AND RESTORE!

Romans 8:5–13

[5]Those who live according to the flesh have their minds set on what the flesh desires; but those who live in accordance with the Spirit have their minds set on what the Spirit desires. [6]The mind governed by the flesh is death, but the mind governed by the Spirit is life and peace. [7]The mind governed by the flesh is hostile to God; it does not submit to God's law, nor can it do so. [8]Those who are in the realm of the flesh cannot please God.

[9]You, however, are not in the realm of the flesh but are in the realm of the Spirit, if indeed the Spirit of God lives in you. And if anyone does not have the Spirit of Christ, they do not belong to Christ. [10]But if Christ is in you, then even though your body is subject to death because of sin, the Spirit gives life because of righteousness. [11]And if the Spirit of him who raised Jesus from the dead is living in you,

He who raised Christ from the dead will also give life to your mortal bodies because of His Spirit who lives in you.

[12]Therefore, brothers and sisters, we have an obligation, but it is not to the flesh, to live according to it. [13]For if you live according to the flesh, you will die; but if by the Spirit you put to death the misdeeds of the body, you will live.

TRINITY FOR HEALTH

"I can do all things through Christ who strengthens me. I commit the next seven weeks of my life to establishing my health and prosperity in my Soul Tank, Body Tank, and Spirit Tank. I will do whatever is required of me to do in order to achieve that level of success in all areas of my life. "

____

Your Signature

____

Partner's Signature

"I am the vine, you are the branches. He who abides in me, and I in him, bears much fruit; for without Me you can do nothing. By this My Father is glorified, that you bear much fruit; so you will be my disciples. "—John 15:5, 8

Part 1

Soul Tank

Soul Tank

Root Cause #1Thoughts—What You Think Can Very Well Make You Sick"

"For "God has not given us a spirit of fear, but of power and of love and of a sound mind."—2 Timothy 1:7

Thoughts are the acts or the process of thinking; deliberation, meditation, or reflection.

What is the focus of your thoughts? The mind is where most battles begin. The human mind is incapable of not thinking, at least on the subconscious level, because of the difficulty in defining a "thought" and the impossibility of determining exactly what is happening within the brain and consciousness at any given moment.

You think about whatever your focus is. If you think happy thoughts, joy comes out of you. If you think sad or angry thoughts, then sadness comes out. If you think sickness and disease, sickness comes out. The saying goes like this: "What goes in must come out."

What causes thoughts? A person's daily routine, tasks, and goals cause thoughts. Thoughts are the way you feel, look; understand things, and how you process information.

Creativity of thought grows out of the desire for change. The word *change* has to do with unpredictability; how much or how little is up to you. Do not repeat old thoughts or ways!

Creativity of thought involves a leap of faith and confidence. Faith is the creative process of changing your thinking. Ultimately thinking is a journey not directed by product but by the passage of memories, vision, intensive observation, time, and focus.

The desire for thought change is a process. It is faith in process. Renewing your thoughts takes discipline and is the critical component in becoming a more positive person and experiencing freedom in all areas of thoughts and life. It is a choice!

"My thoughts tend only to plenteousness."—Proverbs 21:5

The greatest single *barrier* to becoming more healthy and free is the *fear in thoughts.* Changing thoughts demands a step into the unknown. Thoughts should not become a slave of the fears of the mind. Held up in captivity by negative deadly thoughts, one should remember to express happy, healthy thoughts. Thoughts have only to remain true to health and well-being by filters in the mind. Personal thoughts are about vision, growth, and change.

"I have the mind of Christ."—1Corinthians 2:16

Stay awake, stay alert, and change no more "stinkin thinkin. "Look, observe, and re-evaluate, and never stop questioning to see if you are using repeatable negative thoughts and views about yourself or circumstances and situations. Change the voice in your head to line up with what God's Word says about you and your health. He says, you are whole and without spot or blemish.

Often, people are not always aware of all the junk that enters into the mind until it is too late. But you can learn to reprogram and rid the junk before it enters by knowing the patterns of "stinkin' thinkin'." Evaluate what has consumed your thoughts. Don't fear making changes, destroying the image, and so on, because your thoughts have a life of their own, and it's up to you to determine your destiny, which is dependent on your own thoughts.

> "For my thoughts are not your thoughts, neither are your ways my ways," declares the Lord. "As the heavens are higher than the earth, so are my ways higher than your ways and my thoughts than your thoughts."—Isaiah 55:8–9

Training your mind to have pleasant thoughts is a conscious effort, and one that has to be done daily. "The subject of your thoughts and pattern of thought is the bait, but the bait withers away, and the reality of the subject-matter is left and the bait—

the subject matter—disappears. The reality is the residue of the subject-matter this residue perhaps has something tenuously to do with what one started with but very often had very little to do with it. "Whatever is left over from the previous thoughts will determine the course of the next thoughts.

The mind should be borne from the emotional intention of predetermined thoughts. You are able to determine negative or positive thoughts throughout the day. It is a choice to have good or bad thoughts; you have the authority and capability to change your thoughts continuously to line up with what God's Word says about your health, wealth, family, marriage, and virtually every area of your life.

Take more risks with your thinking patterns and predetermined thoughts. The outcome of focusing on thought patterns is that you can always change a particular thought as soon as you are aware of it.

Understand and push the elements of thoughts (focus, subject, emotions, feelings, and meditation/prayer). Consider and be inventive within each element—to the role it plays in your thinking and its impact on the content of thoughts.

When focusing on your thoughts, keep asking the simple but profound questions: *"What am I thinking and taking in? What am I putting out in action and words due to the result of my thoughts?* "Seek clarity in your thoughts while enduring circumstances and situations around you.

Thought in this sense tends towards a complete interlocking of image and precise accompaniment to that image, in memory or reaction to a feeling or emotion. Here the sensory creates the image, pattern, and result of a particular thought. Consequently, every thought in the mind alters the destiny of our lives and implications of the end result and what is coming out of the mouth. That is why it is crucial to focus on thoughts at that moment, then you can proactively utilize preventative measures to break those thought patterns. Since we are creatures to habit especially with our own thoughts, it has become a continuous struggle. Repeating affirmations in our thoughts will ensure the hope of making a fresh perspective in the thinking process.

> "And be not conformed to this world: but be ye transformed by the renewing of your mind, that ye may prove what is that good, and acceptable, and perfect, will of God."- Romans 12:2

Thinking is much more immediate language, and much more direct, than the language of words. You must first think a particular thought before it comes out in words. Clarify your thoughts by continually looking and asking about the "nature of predictability."

Invest in your passion. Where do you find your greatest thoughts? Are they in a person, a place, memory, feeling, experience? If you are confident or consistent in what you think, get to a place where you don't feel so comfortable if negative thoughts are your norm and your comfort zone, then you need to get uncomfortable until positive enhanced thinking becomes the norm. Promote (celebrate) the things (ideas) that are more positive, things which are more whole and healing! Every thought has the ability to take its own path, but only you can control that path.

Where a thought stems from is how a thought is birthed, is there a memory, or sensory that stimulates a thought. Thinking isn't just the visual thing that reaches your mind—it's what is behind it and in it. My intent is to change the process in which your thinking begins from, if I can alter the root of the thought and prevent the thought from even enter in, and then the success rate of actual thought change and pattern is far more successful.

Learn to trust, recognize, follow, and push your personal instincts and feelings in thoughts. The act of creating a thought is a kind of ritual. The origins of feelings and emotions and images in existence lie hidden in this mystery of thoughts and our minds. Human creativity reaffirms and mystifies the power of "life." "Life" is the subject and the object of everything God makes. When the act of creation is really successful, the "thought" creates itself. Our thoughts are a vehicle, and a most valid tool. Once created, the "thought" has a life of its own. I want to live and develop and dwell in thoughts that live and give life and health and vitality" that should be the focus and goal of producing healthy whole thoughts that result in health and well-being in our mind, body, and soul.

> "Those who live according to the flesh have their minds set on what the flesh desires; but those who live in accordance with the Spirit have their minds set on what the Spirit desires. The mind governed by the flesh is death, but the mind governed by the Spirit is life and peace. The mind governed by the flesh is hostile to God; it does not submit to God's law, nor can it do so. Those that are in the realm of the flesh cannot please God. "—Romans 8:5–7

The encouraging news with thought is it won't manifest itself unless is confessed with words. Just because you think it doesn't mean you have to say it.

> "Casting down imaginations, and every high thing that exalteth itself against the knowledge of God, and bringing into captivity every thought to the obedience of Christ."-2nd Corinthians 10:5

Something to Ponder:

With every thought, you have the power to take captive or receive it. You decide the thoughts you want to become flesh. Each thought has to go somewhere; either trash it or let it become life.

Action Item:

Practice thinking about good things every day whenever alone, or have a quiet time. Think happy, healthy, prosperous thoughts that will take root and will manifest themselves. I also encourage reading and spending some time in the Bible, God's Seed that enables good thoughts to enter in.

Words of Affirmation:

I will only think healthy joyful successful thoughts. Any other thought that tries to come into my mind, I will not receive it.

Scripture:

> "As for you, my son Solomon, know the God of your father, and serve Him with a loyal heart and with a willing mind; for the LORD searches all hearts and understands all the intent of the thoughts."—1 Chronicles 28:9

Soul Tank

Root Cause #2—Words, Power of Suggestion

"And God said, 'Let there be light' and there was light."—Genesis 1:3

It has taken me several years to really grasp this system. Most anything in life when successful has had some kind of a system, whether in business, church, or schools. For example, the main reason for fast food chains abundant success is not because they have the best food but because of their proven system that works. That system is duplicated in every location around the world.

The system of the Kingdom of God is the only system that will never fail, go in to debt, fall, crash, or run out of resources. This information I am going to share with you is life changing and worth its weight in gold. Everything on earth was already established in the Spirit. We as humans are three in one, just like God is three in one: the Father, Son and the Holy Spirit. We are spirits that possess a soul and live in a physical body. If everything was first spirit before it was flesh, then the only way for it to manifest is with words, speak it. You have creative ability with your words.

The Kingdom System

- Spirit—Already established, in the unseen reality
- Knowledge of it
- Speak it—words
- Receive it
- Plant it
- Conceive it
- Birth it
- Harvest time

Knowledge of the concept, thing, or idea came first. Then God spoke it into existence. Fruit was then produced and harvest came. In other words, that which was spoken of God was manifested. It was never based on feelings or emotions; it is has always been through the alignment of words spoken equivalent with the Word of God (the Seed).

Since the beginning words have been spoken and manifested in His presence. The Word of God was spoken, and immediately it came to pass. Looking back to the beginning of time and man, it all came about due to the words God spoke.

You are created in the image of Christ. (In the Bible, Jesus says that we shall do greater works than His.)Your very words can shape your life! Those very words have a large impact on your own destiny for your health and well-being!

Think of it this way: there is power in words. You can tell someone you love them with words, as well as tell them you hate them with words. Depending on the words spoken, determines the outcome of the situation.

Thoughts and words obviously go hand in hand. As you think a particular thought the words come out. However, it is critical that the words you speak add life and health, not death and destruction.

"Watch your manner of speech if you wish to develop a peaceful state of mind. Start each day by affirming peaceful, contented and happy words and your days will tend to be pleasant and successful. "—Norman Vincent Peale

Most of the time people don't even consider the words that they speak. They say things out of habit and often let emotions and feelings dictate most, if not all, of their words. Take a moment to digest what you're feeling before you blurt something out. Remember your words are life for your health, finances, marriage, and career.

The next time someone asks you how you are feeling, say something out of the ordinary. The common response is usually, "fine" or "great." Catch them off guard and say something like this: "If I do any better it would be illegal!" Of course, don't forget to smile with the response.

Your body language has a lot to do with your words and the emotions behind your words. If you are feeling down and sickly, you have a tendency to walk hunched over, head down, with a frown on your face. Make up your mind that every day you are going to express joy in your body language and smile. Your words will have to follow in all areas of life: health, finances, marriage, and career. Look at your body language with your marriage as well, because when your marriage is going well, it seems to make a difference in your health and overall well-being.

How often do you encourage yourself or others? Do you constantly go out of your way to do so, or do you avoid the situation all together? Attitude plays an important role in your words. If your attitude is always negative about your health, and you're constantly saying how bad you feel, then your health will start to reflect those words. If you say I feel great, have tons of energy, better than ever, daily you will eventually manifest those emotions and physical attributes. This is the daily renewing of your mind and words.

> "Do not conform to the pattern of this world, but be transformed by the renewing of your mind. Then you will be able to test and approve what God's will is; His good, pleasing and perfect will. "—Romans 12:1–2

In the Bible there are affirmations and declarations of God's perfect Word. His Word is never changing and will never return empty. Since this is a book on spiritual healing as well as physical healing, it only makes sense to go first to the Word of God and see what He says about a circumstance or situation. If God's Word says it, it is already done. By His stripes we have been healed. No weapon formed against you shall prosper. Greater is He that is in you and me than he that is in the world.

Even nonbelievers are in favor of positive language, with several thousand books and teachings on the subject. There are many motivational speakers that teach on this and devoted their entire careers to positive affirmations of words: Anthony Robbins, Zig Ziegler, and Dan Tracy, just to name a few of the best. Although some are worldly based in thought process, they do follow scriptural principals. I have studied and listened too many of these teachings. Much of their advice is to look into a mirror and say things like "I am a good person." "I have a lot to offer." "I am successful, I am pretty, I am thin." Whatever the issue is at the time, you are to affirm yourself with healthy, positive words and declarations over your lives and family, including health and wealth.

Don't Take Words For Granted

They are so easily transported out of the mouth that you do not take the time to really contemplate what should or should not be said or heard. Everyone has wished at one time or another that they could take back what they spoke. If you asked people if they had a time machine, what would they go back and fix, many of them would say the words they spoke to a person regarding a situation.

How many words are spoken in a second, or in a minute? A baby's first words are usually, "mama" or "dada." When we had our children, can you imagine if we started to pump in positive words like, "good boy, you are wonderful," "you are a joy to be around," "you are smart," "you are able to do all things through Christ," and so on. If everyone one of us spoke to our children like that daily we would have a healthy generation of kids and adults and society. What would happen if we started teaching the Word of God to them: "by His stripes you are healed," "Jesus is God," "you can do all things through Christ who strengthens you," "nothing is impossible with God," and so on. What kind of future generation would we have? Words are a key impact to lives in general daily living.

Remember that familiar saying from *Different Strokes* when Arnold would say infamously, "What you talkin' about, Willis?"We all laughed at that dialogue when Arnold realized that Willis had said something foolish or ridiculous. How many moments in time do we say that exact same thing, when we encounter something that was said to us in a foolish or ridiculous manner.

Happy Words Produce Happy Days

We sing praise to God, which is of course just a series of words in harmony to the Lord. However, these are uplifting, encouraging, praiseworthy lyrics. "Speak now or forever hold your peace."Sound familiar? This is what the pastor says right before the groom kisses the bride in a wedding. Other than in a movie, have you ever heard someone say to stop the wedding? "Speak now or forever hold your peace."I really think this is what we really should pay more attention to. Holding our peace can make all the difference in the outcome of many circumstances or situations. Instead of wishing you could take your words back, simply wait and think over what you are about to say and make sure you use your words properly. The end results will be different, and in most cases it will be far better. See scriptures: Exodus 14:14, Job 13:5.

You Are What You Speak

If you continually say negative things about yourself and your health, marriage, or finances, then you will have exactly what you speak of. To prophesy over someone, means to speak forth into their lives about the future. A prophecy is a divine prediction: a prediction of a future event that is believed to reveal the will of God. Prophecy is that which is declared by a prophet in the form of an instruction or an exhortation. God has given us a way to authenticate a prophet and his prophecy: "But a prophet who presumes to speak in God's name anything He has not commanded him to say, or a prophet who speaks in the name of other gods, must be put to death. "Speaking over someone's life is very serious, and it can be a matter of life and death to them and to you. Therefore, speaking over your own life is also prophecy, and again speaking either life or death.

In the book of Matthew, Jesus cursed the fig tree, because it did not produce fruit, and after He spoke the fig tree was barren.

> "Say unto this mountain be thou removed and do not doubt in your heart and it shall be done and cast into the sea."—Matthew 21:18–22

A choice is to be made. Are you going to speak life or death over yourself and others? Are you putting a label on yourself and others in a positive manor or a negative manor? It will make all the difference in the way you look and feel on a daily basis.

Curses or Blessings

Speak blessings: A blessing, (also used to refer to bestowing of such) is the infusion of something with holiness, spiritual, redemption, divine will, or one's hope or approval. There are three

New Testament Greek words related directly to the English word "blessing."

1. *Eulogeitos is* an adjective meaning "well-spoken of; praised. "
2. *Eulogew* is a verb meaning "to speak well of; to praise; to call down God's gracious power. "
3. *Eeulogia* is the noun form, meaning "praise; fine speaking."

So, among Greek-speaking Jews, this was a common word for praise, thanksgiving, and respect. In the King James Version the word "Bless" appears 127 times; the word "blessed" appears 302 times; the word "blessedness" appears 3 times; the word "blesses" appears 3 times; the word "blesseth" appears 8 times; the word "blessing" appears 67 times; the word "blessings" appears 12 times.

> "I will make you into a great nation and I will bless you; I will make your name great, and you will be a blessing. I will bless those who bless you, and whoever curses you I will curse; and all peoples on earth will be blessed through you. "—Genesis 12:2–3

> "If you fully obey the Lord your God and carefully follow all His commands I give you today, the Lord your God will set you high above all the nations on earth. All these blessings will come upon you and accompany you if you obey the

Lord your God: you will be blessed in the city and blessed in the country. The fruit of your womb will be blessed, and the crops of your land and the young of your livestock, the calves of your herds and the lambs of your flocks. Your basket and your kneading trough will be blessed. You will be blessed when you come in and blessed when you go out. The Lord will grant that the enemies who rise up against you will be defeated before you. They will come at you from one direction but flee from you in seven. The Lord will send a blessing on your barns and on everything you put your hand to. The Lord your God will bless you in the land he is giving you. The Lord will establish you as his holy people, as he promised you on oath, if you keep the commands of the Lord your God and walk in his ways. Then all the peoples on earth will see that you are called by the name of the Lord, and they will fear you. The Lord will grant you abundant prosperity in the fruit of your womb, the young of your livestock and the crops of your ground, in the land He swore to your forefathers to give you. The Lord will open the heavens, the storehouse of his bounty, to send rain on your land in season and to bless all the work of your hands. You will lend too many nations but will borrow from none. The Lord will make you the head, not the tail. If you pay attention to the commands of the Lord your God that I give you this day and carefully follow them, you will always be at the top, never at the bottom. Do not turn aside from any of the commands I give you today, to the right or to the left, following other gods and serving them. "—Deuteronomy 28:1–12

Speaking curses is an appeal or prayer for evil or misfortune to befall someone or something.

1. The evil or misfortune coming in or as if in response to such an appeal
2. One that is accursed
3. A source or cause of evil; a scourge
4. A profane word or phrase; a swearword

The relationship of Ahab and Jezebel provides an excellent illustration of the curse brought about by a husband and wife being out of God's divine order for the family. This curse can be traced back all the way to Adam and Eve. It can be found through the Bible being manifested in different families.

We all live with the results of our actions. Blessings are the result of obeying God. Curses are the result of disobeying God.

Curses found in the Bible:

Exodus 34:6–7—Iniquity of fathers on the children
Num. 14:18, 33—Children wandered for 40 years

Deut. 5:9–10—Idol worship

Joshua 24:19–20—serving strange gods

I Kings 21:29—In son's days, evil will come on his house

Job 10:14—Visiting mine iniquity

Psalms 79:8—Remember not against us former iniquities

Isaiah 64:9—Neither remembers iniquity forever

In Christ's Kingdom, children of the Most High God are far removed from curses. The blessings are so much on us, it is impossible to think any other way. Because of the precious blood that was shed, we can abide in blessings and no longer under the curses. We will dive more into generational curses later in this book.

Speak faith building, confident, encouraging, life giving, healthy words in every area of your life. You can choose to begin today!

Something to Ponder

1. There is power in the tongue; you choose what goes out of your mouth; is it life or death?
2. Blessings or curses, love or hate? You will choose your destiny just by the words spoken out of your own mouth. Speak your words wisely.

Action Item

If you need to create a new habit of life-giving words, look in a mirror and practice saying seven positive words about health every day, then seven positive words about your family members every day. Do this for two months without missing a day and you will soon see those words manifest in your life. It works!

Next Steps—Word of Affirmation

"I am happy, full of joy, healthy, prosperous, and full of vitality and I lack no good thing in my life nothing missing, nothing wanted, nothing needed, nothing broken."

Scripture

> "My son, attend to my words, incline thy ears to my sayings. Let them not depart from thine eyes; keep them in the midst of thine heart; for they are life to those that find them and health to all their flesh. "—Proverbs4:20–23

Christ's words have power in them and your own words also have power in them. You are to be like Christ and do as Christ has done. He spoke it, and it was so; now it is up to His children.

Since every conceivable thing, idea, concept, provision, wholeness and any possible need is already established and deposited in you, your only job is to have faith. Speak the words to see it manifest, and enjoy the harvest of your faith-filled words.

Soul Tank

Root Cause #3—Spiritual Houses

Who's moving in?

Do you ever just feel overwhelmed and weighed down with the cares of life? Maybe you are more tired than normal, or you just feel blah. There are days when I just can't put my finger on it. These days are very few lately, but in the past I had many of them.

One spring day after taking a cat nap, I got to thinking that life is all about choices, right and wrong. Pondering back nine years, I asked myself, "What if?"If I hadn't gone to the restaurant that day, I never would have met my husband, had my amazing son, or would even be writing this book. If I hadn't met my husband, I never would have started the business. I would never have received the loan from his investor, and the rest as they say, is history.

Imagine the most spectacular times in your life; they were derived from a choice you made. You said "yes" to someone or something, or in some cases maybe you said "no. " If you had said "yes" when you should have said "no," or went somewhere else, or did something else, your life would have a different spin on it. Maybe a new direction or path in life would have occurred. That is either a good thing or a bad thing depending, of course, on the situation.

I have come to the conclusion that all those choices, whether right or wrong, and the consequences from each choice, are what we live with. If it is a wrong choice, then the results of the choices could have been traumatic, and the results are soul wounds. The same goes for right choices; the end result is victories. As these experiences transpire and we store the emotional, physical, and spiritual consequences in our lives, they become one with us. When that oneness takes place, then those possessions go into our spiritual houses, tanks, or vessels.

We all have spiritual houses to store stuff. These are houses that we all possess, and they are not brick and mortar; they are our holding tanks, both spiritual and physical vessels. It's like any other brick and mortar house we move into; our lives are poured into our houses. We move in our furniture, baggage from the old house, pictures, knick knacks, and all our valuable and invaluable items. We do our best to make it comfortable and our own place of refuge and escape.

We may have way too much stuff for our houses and end up with storage units for the extra things we have accumulated, such as the treadmill we had to have, the $300 juicer we never opened, jewelry, extra furniture, and so on. If we have all this extra stuff for our brick and mortar houses we live in, how much extra stuff is in our spiritual houses? No, not furniture, but definitely old baggage, past relationships, hurt feelings, negative thoughts, and unforgiveness. Our spiritual houses are our mind, body, and soul. Each one of these houses has storage facilities (holding tanks) for all the extra stuff we really don't need but continue to hold on to. According to an article published in the Washington Post, we are occupying an average of 24% per capita share of the Great American Self Storage Empire. According to the Self Storage Association, a trade group charged with monitoring such things, the country now possesses some 1. 875 billion square feet of personal storage space. All this space is contained in nearly 40,000 facilities.

Not only do we store stuff, we store other people's stuff as well. When a relationship begins, you get to know that person and learn of all their bad and good habits, such as whether they were married before and the ex and kids if they have any, their weaknesses, and their strengths. If that relationship develops and there is sexual intimacy, you now have a soul tie. When God said to procreate he meant it for reproducing life, not just to sleep with everyone we meet. When a person becomes one with someone sexually there is a vow between them, and their souls become tied together. If that relationship ends, not only do you have your own baggage from that relationship, but now you also have the baggage of that other person. You have unknowingly become a storage facility of negativity, self-condemnation, anger, sadness, frustration, depression, unforgiveness, and so much other drama. You bring not only your own stuff into your storage tanks, but you also carry the burdens of other people's spiritual tanks. Why do you feel the need to take in other peoples junk when you can barely handle our own junk? It is because of the bond that develops in that relationship, not just with spouses but in all relationships where we genuinely care for that person.

Dissecting each of these examples, you will see the cause and effect of toxic spiritual houses: negative thoughts, cursing tongue, gossip, anger, jealousy, greed, lust, perversion, blasphemy, fear, disobedience, unforgiveness, witchcraft, manipulation, and guilt to name a few.

In an actual brick and mortar house we lock our doors, and set alarms to keep thieves out. In the spiritual house our door is always open and never shut, unless you have keen discernment. It can be difficult to tell when a thief is going to enter in the spiritual house, and the only alarm to warn is the Holy Spirit. Many times it is too late; the damage is already done. Unless you are being led by the spirit and not the flesh, you can fall victim to false identities and their toxic spiritual houses. People can just come in and dump all their personal garbage on you, and once you receive it, it becomes very difficult to release. Many times you have emotional connections to the garbage that is dumped, and you try to help,

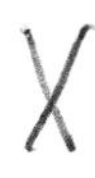

not realizing it is stored in us as well. We have connections to a lot of different people, and all the stuff they bring with them into our houses. They just move right in, and usually it is more than just a brief visit. They become the guests that wouldn't leave.

So how do we proceed in life with all this junk we have in our houses?

One of the amazing mercies of our God is that you are forgiven of all your sins, and they are remembered no more. It doesn't matter what you have done in the past; mistakes, failures, hurts. All that matters is you have a new beginning, and it is holy and blameless and full of God's amazing unconditional love. You need to know it all began with Christ's love for you. He created you out of love, gave you all things out of love, and His Son's blood was shed for your sins, all out of love. His love consumes you, like a volcano that is ready to erupt always, never ending, with hot lava covering over your entire being. His love is a fire consuming you; His love is never-ending and never fails. So the answer to living in a storage free house is Jesus. It doesn't matter what you have done; it is where you are headed and what your house looks like going forward.

Root Cause #4—Spiritual Accounts

Lock Boxes

Not only do we have spiritual houses, but we also have spiritual bank accounts. This bank account is always full; there is no lack whatsoever, and it is always ready to pay out. We never have to get a loan; these accounts are fully accessible; there is abundance wherever we go.

Unlike our own bank accounts, unfortunately, the only time we can withdraw is after we made deposits, and most of us have to work many hours in jobs we may not like but simply are enduring to put food on the table and make those deposits. Subsequently, in most cases there have been overdrawn accounts, nonsufficient funds, and bad checks written. There have been many occasions in my own checking account when it went negative due to negligence on my behalf and not balancing my checkbook correctly. I have also made some very careless purchases that had contributed to my disobedience within my own spending habits and miscalculating what I actually had in my accounts. I remember on several occasions I didn't have enough to cover payroll, and only through the grace of God was I able to pay my employees on time. This is not the case, however, in our spiritual bank account. We never have lack, and there is never a negative balance in any of our spiritual bank accounts. If you don't have God, this is could become your harvest.

Along with the houses and bank accounts, many of us also have safe deposit boxes or as I like to call them, lock boxes: storage facilities maintained in the vault area of a bank that is rented to customers for safekeeping of personal valuables, such as birth and marriage certificates, passports, jewelry, and other valuable items. These lock boxes are hardly ever used.

We make deposits into our lock boxes without realizing it. We have a mind lock box (thoughts), will lock box (bad habits) and emotions lock box (feelings) and of course a flesh lock box (lymphatic system and digestive system).

EMOTIONAL LOCK BOX

An emotional lock box is extremely full and constantly has deposits daily, by the choices we make. However, it is not being withdrawn from very often; it just becomes a safekeeping storage box with a special key. An example of a deposit in your lock box: if you have an argument with your spouse and it is right before an event, you are going to be around a lot of people, and this is not the time to argue about it in detail. So you store up the feelings that you are experiencing at the time of the fight, and you keep them for later. Then after the event you go home, and the kids are all around you, so you can't let those feeling out yet. Again you store or bottle those emotions up, and by this time it is getting more and more intense because you can't release what is in you. The next day you and your spouse are bogged down with work; life goes on, and you just end up saying, "Oh forget it, it's not even worth mentioning it anymore. "That is one example of a lock box deposit. Think about how many of those types of deposits are going into each one of your lock boxes: mind, will, emotions, and flesh boxes. You are storing what should be released and eliminated.

That argument you had is buried and rooted deep inside you; hence the emotional lock box it is put away safely until it gets purged, or emptied out when you explode at any time and at any place. When it releases, it goes into the emotional bank account, no longer in the lock box, but now it is available for withdrawals.

PHYSICAL LOCK BOX

You may eat your meals daily; maybe snack occasionally, drink coffee, smoke cigarettes, take medications. If you do this continually for months or even years, a pattern starts to develop, and the body goes into survival mode and stores what is necessary and needed. Where do you think it all goes? We all know when you digest food it goes into the mouth and into the stomach. That is all that most people know. The digestive system comprises the digestive tract (starting from the mouth and ending at the anus) and several other organs that help in the digestion process. The organs of the digestive tract are mouth, esophagus, stomach, intestine (small and large), and anus. During the process of digestion, the mucosa lining of the mouth, stomach, and small intestine secretes enzymes that aid in the digestion of food.

The smooth muscle lining of the digestive tract also helps in the mechanical breakdown of the food. The organs, liver, and pancreas produce digestive juices or enzymes that help in breaking down the complex food substances (fats and lipids) into simpler forms. If you don't eliminate on a daily basis, the digestive system becomes clogged and immobile and is not able to function or release properly.

Unfortunately not very many people have eliminated daily, without fail, since birth. Yet our bodies were designed by God, whole and perfect, and meant to eliminate daily. There is a missing equation here with what goes in and what comes out. It doesn't really add up. We seem to take in way more food and toxins than our body's ability to eliminate; it gets stagnant and becomes sluggish.

The lymphatic's function (remember the lymphatic system is also part of the physical lock box) is the holding tank for garbage. It is literally a garbage disposal for toxins and fat. All the food and leftover waste that has not been eliminated goes in that system. A healthy system filters out organisms that cause disease, produces certain white blood cells, and generates antibodies. It is also important for the distribution of fluids and nutrients in the body, because it drains excess fluids and protein so that tissues do not swell up. "Lymph" is a milky body fluid that contains a type of white blood cells, called "lymphocytes," along with proteins and fats. Lymph seeps outside the blood vessels in spaces of body tissues and is stored in the "lymphatic" system to flow back into the bloodstream. Through the flow of blood in and out of arteries, and into the veins, and through the lymph nodes and into the lymph, the body is able to eliminate the products of cellular breakdown and bacterial invasion of toxic waste.

The most unfortunate issue is that many people have unhealthy blocked up lymphatic systems that don't allow the release of lymph fluid to excrete out. So they end up becoming toxic waste dumps. The complimentary partner of the lymphatic system is the digestive system. Both systems (Physical Lock Box) play very important roles in the overall health and prosperity of the soul. This lock box is not a choice of yours to deposit in. This lock box is your survival and doesn't always allow you to withdraw when you want to.

You are the only one who has the keys to those boxes. Although the enemy thinks he has a right into those boxes, it is only when you allow him. He is chomping at the bit for you to open up those boxes, full of past hurts, bad choices, negative thoughts and feelings, unforgiveness, anger, hidden addictions and patterns, and soul wounds. He knows about your past wounds and hovers around waiting to peak his head in. Remember only Jesus knows you intimately. The enemy only knows the weakness of the flesh.

All the past wounds and traumas that have happened to you since you were born are in those boxes. You most likely won't remember many of those since you may have a tendency to have a selective memory with past junk. But it is in there, buried beneath other things that are still there. Your past wounds have been stored up; you continue to make deposits. The question is, what kind of deposits are you making?

MIND LOCK BOX

The mind lock box (thoughts) is the most dangerous and deadly of them all. It also can be the most fruitful and healthy of them all. Everything starts in the mind; if you are hungry, tired, sick, happy, sad, or angry, it all begins with a thought. Your attitude begins with a thought. Your decisions begin with a thought. You are programmed with thoughts by your loved ones since birth. You either have deposits of healthy and edifying thoughts or negative, destructive thoughts. The mind lock box and the flesh lock box are very complimentary, in that the mind has a lot to do with the deposits of the flesh lock box. Also in this lock box you have memories of events and thoughts generated throughout the years.

When you remember something, your mind will "travel back in time" to the moment and circumstance when you formed that memory. Memory functions can be described in the following way: When you are in a certain situation, certain things may attract your attention and generate emotions, thoughts, and feelings. When you are recalling something, you may revisit your imagination in that certain situation, and the brain generates the same emotions, thoughts, and feelings.

WILL LOCK BOX

Directly connected to the mind lock box is the will lock box (bad habits). After certain thoughts or memories surface, many times the will lock box comes to play. You may begin to form bad habits, like running away from conflict, swearing, expressing anger, drinking heavily, or taking drugs. It is your own attitudes from your thoughts and emotions that dictate your behavior and deposits in the will lock box.

Rebellion is a big deposit. We all make choices; right and wrong choices will determine your fate. This lock box has a lot to do with the way you handle those choices. Another deposit is disobedience, the sister of rebellion and very unpleasing to the Lord. You are to be an obedient servant to your Heavenly Father.

SPIRITUAL BANK ACCOUNT

You can only withdraw what you deposit. So, in essence, we all have our own bank accounts, and none of us are going bankrupt. There is always plenty of activity going in the accounts. What are your deposits, and who are your depositors and withdrawers? They are anyone or anything that cause issues to be deposited, like loved ones, enemies, loss of a job, a physical injury, hurt feelings, a disappointment, past sins. Even your own loved ones are depositors in your accounts, in your jobs, in your financial situations, in your physical and emotional falls, bumps and bruises. You have different accounts for each area of the soul (mind, will, and emotions), and your body, which is the end result of the condition of your spiritual bank. Your lock boxes are the vaults that are locked and forgotten about. The accounts have daily activity and constantly have deposits and withdrawals.

MIND

The mind account is negative thoughts. It begins with a small deposit, but this is the fullest account out of all of them. When you were born, you were told not to touch this and don't do that. The negative mind account began. That account is one of the first accounts to be opened. You never really look in your vault's deposits, but they are always there and ready for action.

WILL

The will account is the stubborn, rebellious account. When you were little you may have said, "Oh yeah, I'll show you, I am going to touch that thing you told me not to, I am going to say that thing you said not to say, and I am going to do what I know you said I can't do. "This account has no lack either; this is where many of your choices become realities, not just thoughts anymore. Many withdrawals come out of this account. Deposits are made more in the mind account; the will account is a withdrawal-only account. These two accounts are joint accounts, the mind and will accounts.

EMOTIONS

The emotional bank accounts have many deposits and withdrawals, equal amounts in each. This account is a cause and effect account. If someone does good to you, you give out good. When someone does badly to you, you dish out bad. These accounts are hard to lock away in lock boxes because they are always right there in the open. You have a debit card for this account. Many times you may like to just deposit, store, and forget about all your past deposits. However, the emotions are right there ready for release as well, whenever the urge hits you. It is a two-in-one bank account and lock box account. Whenever you need to pull out an emotion, there it is, ready to go with a quick debit card withdrawal. The joint account to this is the flesh (body) account. Just have someone do you wrong, and your flesh takes over, and you go to town. Many times the deposits of the emotional account carry over to the flesh account. It's like an insufficient funds account; if there isn't enough in one it automatically goes into the other.

FLESH

The flesh account (physical body account) is the most visible account for all to see on display. This account shows any lack in your body, such as sickness or disease. You can see most of your emotional, mind, and will choices of withdrawals and deposits in your flesh. You make choices; what you say and do, and how healthy your body is, is the end result of your spiritual flesh account. This is the fullest account available. Much of the mind, will, and emotional accounts manifest in your flesh account.

CHANGING ACCOUNTS

So what happens when you want to change bank accounts and close one out? It is possible, but real work inside has to be done. A lot of healing and cleansing has to take place in those accounts. You need to clear out all deposits and flush the accounts. The way to do that is to reprogram your mind, forgive others, break all soul ties and generational curses, and make a choice to say, "Yes" to God and "No" to everything else.

> "Be not conformed to the ways of the world, but be transformed to the renewing of your mind that ye may prove what is that good, and acceptable, and perfect, will of God "—Romans 12: 2

It is only then that you will begin to see the manifestation of those bank accounts changing deposits and withdrawals. Remember you can only get out what is put in.

For true revelation and change, you first must have ownership in your mind of the healing to take place. Once this is established as a part of your being in your soul account, you will see it manifested in your flesh account. But there is a definite developing and a processing that must be inherited prior to manifestation of the flesh account. This is where the meat of it happens; if you have an easy time believing in the bad stuff in your mind and it takes root, after a while it will take its place in manifesting in the flesh account and mind account.

The same is true when you have a positive life-changing mind set. The first account that needs to change is the mind account. Since you have most deposits in that account, the most cleansing and clearing out has to take place. You have deep seated deposits of memories in your accounts and lock boxes. From birth to adulthood you take mental notes of those things, storing them in your lock box accounts.

With a divorce or a loss of a loved one, feelings and emotions get deposited immediately in your emotional accounts. As time goes by those feelings and memories are stored in the lock box with all the other past deposits. Whenever there is a fresh feeling, emotion, or experience good or bad, they go in to the appropriate accounts—an instant deposit. After awhile those feelings have gone by the wayside; you don't remember them much, so they go into the lock box for safekeeping. They are still there ready to be accessed at any time, which is why old songs can trigger good and bad emotions.

Your lock boxes can be full and overflowing, with no lack in them. When you have regret, you hold grudges, unforgiveness, and hurt feelings that are triggered when you see someone you haven't seen for many years. Those old feelings surface just as if the triggering event happened yesterday.

There is another phase your accounts go into: they can be active or dormant. The active accounts are having deposits made on a regular basis. The dormant accounts are stagnant. Maybe you are overdrawn on your accounts and you want to close out those accounts, but you have no idea how. You know they are causing you more problems, and you need to stop all deposits and withdrawals. Maybe you were successful in closing some accounts. Maybe you are making new deposits, more positive deposits. Well, how long will that last, until another negative emotion triggers an old deposit that is stored up in the lock box? Constant, daily reprogramming of putting in good healthy deposits in all your accounts and ridding yourself of the negative lock boxes in your spiritual bank accounts is required. Focus on what you put in and take out in all your spiritual accounts so that you become healthy billionaires in your own banks. How do you become billionaires in your own accounts?

We have all been designed to be like Christ, made in His image, bone of His bone, flesh of His flesh. Most of us know that because we were taught that when we were kids in Bible school, or from our parents. But when you truly understand what that means, it will amaze you at the simplicity of it all. This revelation will actually assist in the deliverance from many addictions.

Everyone at one time or another has had a yearning for more: more stuff, more love, more money, more happiness, more, more, and even more! You were created by God; He is your maker, your author and finisher, and He gives you the desires of your heart. You were created to pursue and seek only Him and you were designed to want more, more of Him. Because of the desire for more, you may have turned to food, drugs, alcohol, and sex, whatever you could get that filled you up. You experience lack because you were designed to want more, but the more of what you were designed for is more of God. Only God can satisfy the hunger in you. The craving for drugs, alcohol, and sex is all because the desire for more was manufactured in you from the beginning of time, and you were born with it in the womb, and it kept developing as you grew.

If you were not getting the spiritual food you desired and craved, you may have tried to satisfy the hunger in any way possible. It was not physical food, material things, worldly success, or satisfaction you needed. It was the bread of life you needed to be satisfied and completely filled.

You may have searched for that total void to be filled in many ways, with no success and with only disappointment. You didn't find it in relationships because you tried to be filled up by others and with their approval but found it an impossible pursuit. You were not created to please men, but to please God. You may have craved love and praise of others, even though you may have had the love of your parents. You may still be searching for it, but you will realize only God can give you what you are lacking or missing in life. This is when you will have peace that surpasses all understanding and unspeakable joy; it is not predicated on possessions, people, places or things but only in God the Father, Holy Spirit, and Jesus the Son.

You have all you need in your bank accounts and in your lock boxes just by the spiritual food, love, wisdom, and care God has for you. Only God can fill you up and satisfy your every need, and only He can reprogram your deposits and withdrawals. It is impossible for us to do it all on our own; only God can change what needs to be changed for your accounts and lock boxes.

Something to Ponder:

Who and what are moving into your house and how long are you going to let unwanted guests stay where they are not welcome?

What do your accounts look like?

Are they withdrawal only, or are they deposit only? The choice is yours.

Action Item:

Take inventory of all unwanted storage in your spiritual house. Look in all your accounts and lock boxes, and see what you are putting in and taking out of each of them. Write a list of every thought, word or memory that is full of waste, and eliminate them as you go through your house and rid it of unwanted baggage.

Words of Affirmation:

All my houses are cleansed and my bank accounts are prosperous.

Scripture:

> "Now may He who supplies seed to the sower, and bread for food, supply and multiply the seed you have sown and increase the fruits of your righteousness. "—2 Corinthians 9:10

Root Cause #5—Sin and Disobedience

The world was created through the Word spoken by God. The world was manifested from a spiritual realm that was already there. The human eye was not able to see it until it became manifested physically. Everything was spirit before it was physical. We are a spirit; we possess a soul, and live in a physical body.

If there is an understanding of spirit and physical body (or flesh) then there can be revelation of what sin is and how it began. Due to sin, there is sickness and death. With the understanding of this you can begin to see how it is possible to overcome all health challenges in the body and soul.

The World's System of Sickness and Disease

If we know the formula at the beginning of sickness, then we can also know the solution to the formula in reestablishing health.

- ❖ Sickness enters physical body, due to sin
- ❖ Pain or discomfort is experienced through the physical senses
- ❖ Words spoken affirm pain or discomfort
- ❖ Immediate pain or confusion sets in
- ❖ Treatment is sought
- ❖ Treatment begins
- ❖ Potential side effects take place
- ❖ More words are spoken confirming side effects
- ❖ Additional treatment is sought
- ❖ Potential and additional side effects take place, and so on . . .
- ❖ Sickness progresses
- ❖ Sickness wins

As you look at this formula, it is almost humorous that it is done every day, by millions of people.

Let's look at the way the Kingdom of God treats sickness and disease.

- ❖ Sickness enters into the physical body
- ❖ Body starts to feel it (in the senses)
- ❖ Words begin, speaking against the sickness
- ❖ Confirming God's promise, by His stripes you are healed
- ❖ Stand on the Word, immovable
- ❖ Doctor says something negative
- ❖ Doctor prescribes drugs

- ❖ Don't accept sickness or drug
- ❖ Continue to stand on the Word
- ❖ Healed completely; Gods Word is true
- ❖ Health wins

What is Sin?

Sin is the transgression of theological principles: an act, thought, or way of behaving that goes against the law or teachings of a religion, especially when the person who commits it is aware of this. It is a knowing of what is right and wrong. It is an understanding of an act of disobedience against the commands of God.

Jesus died for our sins, so what have we been saved from? When we say "yes" to Jesus, and "no" to our own fleshly desires and ways, we enter into a covenant of salvation with all the benefits. We have been saved from ourselves and our own wicked ways.

This is foolproof only when you accept Christ into your life; then you have received the forgiveness of sins. Until that acceptance you are still walking around in spiritual darkness and not realizing the gift that was given to you. Your sins are already forgiven; you just don't know it. If you have never asked Christ to be your Lord and Savior, now is the perfect time. Jesus gave His life for your iniquities; the price was already paid; He exchanged curses for blessings, just for you.

Just because a person believes (or does not believe) does not make this true or false; God's Word and work on the cross is finished and is true. It is already established. It does not change and will not return void. Many people act as if they have some sort of say in the matter of the realm of the Kingdom of God. But it is finished, whether people choose to believe or not. It is so exciting to know that all I have to do is come to Christ, and He has everything already worked out for me. He works behind the scenes, preparing the way, just for me.

My personal definition of sin is any word, thought, or deed that goes against the written and spoken Word of God. In the Book of Matthew, verse 6:25, God says to have no thought about food, clothing, or shelter. People worry about those things and try and operate outside of God's Kingdom by thinking that worry is faith. They are operating in doubt and disbelief, which is sin.

Where there is faith, there is no fear. Walking in faith is more easily said than done, but God's Word is truth, and it cannot and will not return to Him void it cannot fail. Why would you put your hope, expectation and trust in a world that is failing daily?

> "Knowing this, that the old man was crucified with Him so that the body of sin might be done away with; that we should no longer be slaves of sin."—Romans 6:6

Walking with God means no more detours; His will be done on earth as it is in heaven that's what God has declared. We are to live heaven on earth; that means whatever is loosed in heaven is loosed on earth, and whatever is bound in heaven is bound on earth. We are to be the liaison between heaven and earth. I truly believe that it's blasphemy to live any other way. God did not send His only begotten Son to die for us so that we can still suffer in want and need. But it was so we will live a more abundant life!

> "The thief does not come except to steal, and to kill, and to destroy. I have come that they may have life, and that they may have it more abundantly. " John 10:10

The joy and peace of God lives inside you, and God is available to all who will call unto Him and receive Him unto Himself.

If you are reading this book and you don't personally have a relationship with Christ, you can begin right now. Just ask Him to be your Lord and Savior and to come into your heart. He will take you just as you are and cleanse you with His precious blood. Ask him to forgive your sins; without repentance there is no shedding of his blood for you.

The Blood That Cleanses

In the Old Testament they would bring an offering or a sacrifice to the Lord, and it was always with blood. This was their atoning sacrifice of animals for cleansing of their wrongs and iniquities. In the Old Testament they continued to do this every time, over and over again as they would repent for their wrongdoing.

In the New Testament we have Jesus who made the eternal sacrifice, the one-time atonement for all of us and our sins. He brought us back before the fall of man in the Garden of Eden and wiped our sins away, so they are remembered no more, and they were put to death with Him on the cross.

> "Then Jesus said to them, "Most assuredly, I say to you, unless you eat the flesh of the Son of Man and drink His blood, you have no life in you."—John6:53

Putting on the New Man

> "I have been crucified with Christ; it is no longer I who live, but Christ lives in me; and the life which I now live in the flesh I live by faith in the Son of God, who loved me and gave Himself for me."—Galatians2:20

This simply means dying to your flesh, saying no to worldly desires and thoughts and deeds, and saying "Yes" to Christ and His Kingdom.

If you are seeking health and wholeness in every area of your life, then the question to ask is: where is my sin, what is my sin and how can I repent from my sin today? God knows all and sees all anyway; you cannot hide from God or your sin.

Something to Ponder

No matter what you have done, or are presently doing, or where you came from, it is where you are going that matters. Jesus loves you just as you are. We all have the same God, Jesus and Holy Spirit. Our sins have all been forgotten, and there is no memory of any of them. You literally can start over today; all it takes is the choice to do so.

Action Steps

There is only one step to take for this chapter, and that is, if you haven't already done so, give your life to Christ. Ask Him into your life and thank Him for forgiving your sins. If you are saved then now is a good time to recommit to Christ and start reading the word on a daily basis. Your life will never be the same guarenteed.

Words of Affirmation

"I am a child of God, no longer of the world, I am a royal son or daughter of God, I am under the covering and the covenant of Kingdom and free from the sins of the world with access through the blood of Jesus. I am back in the Garden of Eden, before the fall of man. I have a spiritual do-over in my life. "

Scripture

"But now in Christ Jesus ye who sometimes were far off are made nigh by the blood of Christ. "—Ephesians2:13

Root Cause #6—GenerationalCurses

The apple doesn't fall far from the tree.

Generational Curses

Generational curses are defined based on past sins of your parents. Since the Biblical Law is that you will reap what you sow, every defining moment in life is seed, time, and harvest. Whether you are Christian or not, the same applies to everyone.

> "Keeping mercy for thousands, forgiving iniquity and transgression and sin, and that will by no means clear the guilty; visiting (punishing) the iniquity of the fathers upon the children, and upon the children's children, unto the third and to the fourth generations. "—Exodus 34:7

"Our fathers have sinned, and are not; and we have borne (been punished for) their iniquities."—Lamentations 5:7

It only makes sense that generational curses are a root cause for sickness and disease such as alcoholism, drug addiction, and abuse. Doctors have done studies on genetics and say that some diseases are because of family history. When it comes to generational curses, it only makes sense that you become what you are around and what your predominant daily influence is. That is why it is so important to surround yourself with the people you want to become like. Most, if not all, addictions are generational. If you were abused as a child, chances are there will be some kind of abuse in your life, either as a receiver, or as an abuser.

Genetics

Genetics are the DNA in the cells when you were first born; it is a predetermined lineage of your cells from your parents. Some sickness is due to genetic predisposition. Even genetics can be changed and altered to line up with God's holy written and spoken Word. Nothing is impossible with God. By His stripes you are healed; there are no restrictions on God's healing; He is your creator, the author and the finisher of your life (1 Peter 2:24, Isaiah55:6).

Let's look at genetics: what you are born with. You can only have these genetic issues because you had past generations that had the same issues. So if sin causes sickness, and it began there, then genetics started first as a generational curse.

Let's dig into what generational curses are. Curses are in the category of social matters because of their expressive nature. They have to either be spoken or written. Generational means that all of the offspring that are at the same stage of descent from a common ancestor.

The reason future generations were cursed is because they have sinned and continue to live in sin nature. God hates disobedience, rebellion, and sin. We are, in a sense, paying the price because of ancestors in generations past. That is why all generational curses need to end and be destroyed for good.

A curse is any expressed wish that some form of adversity or misfortune will befall or attach to some other entity, or one or more persons, place, or object. In the case of generational curses, it is persons, habits, and choices of that person and the past generations.

Sickness and Generational Curses

If your mother had breast cancer, there is a chance you'll get it since you are a descendant of hers. If you look along your family tree, there could be a history of cancer in your family. So what can you do if it is genetic and from a generational curse?

If you are a believer, you can stop it! You have all the authority to do so. Just because your mother or father had a genetic disposition does not mean it needs to go to you. It can stop with you so you won't continue to pass on the genes, or the curses that plagued your family for decades.

How to Stop Curses or Genetic Genes

The good news is that once you accept Jesus, the transference of bondage stops from your ancestors in the form of generational curses. You can no longer receive spiritual bondages in this manner once you accept Jesus! You can receive them, *but* you can cut yourself loose from them. Christ was made a curse so you can be freed from the curses that sin (both our sins and those of our forefathers) have brought.

> "Christ hath redeemed us from the curse of the law, being made a curse for us: for it is written, 'Cursed is every one that hangeth on a tree. '"—Galatians 3:13

If we don't know, confess, and believe in the Word in our lives, then curses can and will influence lives. Once you become a child of God, no longer will the sins of your parents plague you.

Say "No" to sickness, disease, or genetic issues. Read the Word of God and see what is said about blessings and how children of God are no longer under the curse and that it was done away with through the blood of Jesus. The promise is ours, but like any other promise of God, we must pick up the promises in the Word and stand in authority of the Word of God to drive the enemy out.

Daily Devotional

"Heavenly Father, I thank you and praise Your mighty name that I am no longer under any generational curses. I understand and agree with what your mighty Word says about delivering me from all present and future curses. I continue to declare your blessings upon myself and all that I put my hands to. I thank you that genetics no longer plague me, or my family, in my health and well-being; in Jesus' precious name, amen. "

Something to Ponder

Many times when you could experience sickness or addiction it is because generational curses have not been broken. It is your choice to break them all and have all generational curses stop with you.

Action Item

Go through your genealogy and family history and look at patterns in your family members and also look at any genetic issues the family may have had. Just because they had it does *not* mean you have to. Break all generational curses in the mighty name of Jesus.

Words of Affirmation

"I am free; there are no generational curses in my family. I renounce and break any and all curses from myself and all other family members."

Scripture

> "Do not be deceived: God cannot be mocked. A man reaps what he sows." Galatians 6:7

Root Cause #7—SoulTies

When I was first introduced to "soul ties," I instantly I wanted to break and destroy every last one of them. I wanted to be set free from any souls I had been previously and ignorantly connected with. I wish I was taught about this in my early adolescent years. I know I would have made many different choices.

I was very baffled at the connection of any soul ties; anyone I had any kind of sexual connection with was connected to my soul and a part of me. The Bible says that when a man and woman marry, their flesh becomes one, and they leave parents and cleave to each other.

> "For this cause shall a man leave father and mother, and shall cleave to his wife: and they two shall be one flesh. "—Matthew 19:5

Soul ties can also be used for your enemy's advantage. Soul ties formed from sex outside of marriage, which causes a person to become defiled.

> "And when Shechem the son of Hamor the Hivite, prince of the country, saw her, he took her, and lay with her, and defiled her. And his soul cleaved unto Dinah the daughter of Jacob, and he loved the damsel, and spoke kindly unto the damsel."—Genesis 34:2–3

This is why it is so common for a person to still have "feelings" towards an ex-lover that they have no right to be attracted to. Even twenty years later, a person may still think of their first lover, even if he or she is across the country and has their own family. This can happen because of a soul tie!

Demonic spirits can also take advantage of ungodly soul ties and use them to transfer spirits from one person to another. I remember one young man I led through deliverance. He was facing severe demonic visitations and torment because of an ungodly soul tie. I led him to break the soul tie, and the attacks stopped completely!

> "And the Babylonians came to her into the bed of love, and they defiled her with their whoredom, and she was polluted with them."—Ezekiel 23:17

What constitutes that formality is consummating the marriage vows and making a promise in front of God and that person; to give your selves to each other forever.

Unless you were a virgin when you married, you are connected to all other partners you were intimate with. Now why is that such an issue with your health, and why would it be considered a root cause? It is simple: if you become one with someone else, your souls are now joined and all their soul wounds become your soul wounds. They will affect you, but they don't become yours.

Soul ties can also bring abuse in other relationships. Patterns and addictions in your life, such as drugs, alcohol, and abuse, draw you to the same patterns in anyone you have been intimate with until you become free of the soul ties that brought them in the first place.

Avoiding Other Soul Ties

An example of a soul tie is when a baby is in the womb of the mother, and that baby receives all the nutrients from the mother's food. When the mother eats something with caffeine the baby will respond to it. If the mother is stressed, the baby responds to the stress. Let's say the mother is drinking alcohol or doing drugs; the baby is also doing drinking alcohol or doing drugs. The baby and the mother are one; the connection is the umbilical cord. In order for that connection to be broken the umbilical cord must be cut, so now the baby and the mother are individuals

and able to live completely separate lives.

You have to cut and sever all old ties befor

life. You can see the importance in severing the soulish umb

cord from those you have been within the past. As long as you are connected in the soul with someone from the past, it is difficult to move forward.

Many single people want to get married, but they are not ready because they have to get themselves prepared for the bride or bridegroom. The most important thing is getting rid of the old and allowing the new to come forth. If you go into a marriage with your past not buried and all the ties severed, the memories on your soul will try to bring them back.

> "For though we walk in the flesh, we do not war after the flesh."- 2Corinthians 10:3

> "For the weapons of our warfare are not carnal, but mighty through God to the pulling down of strongholds."—2 Corinthians 10:4

> "Casting down imaginations, and every high thing that exalteth itself against the knowledge of God, and bringing into captivity every thought to the obedience of Christ."—2 Corinthians 10:5

"For we wrestle not against flesh and blood, but against principalities, against powers, against the rulers of the darkness of this world, against spiritual wickedness in high places."—Ephesians 6:12

Breaking Free!

Make a list of soul ties. Identify each soul you have been tied to, sexually, or in any other form or relationship that was unhealthy or destructive. Pray and ask God to bring to your remembrance all the people you have connections with from your childhood; that includes any unhealthy relationships with your parents or siblings or any other family members. This is a process and may not be instantaneous, so be consistent and tenacious. If you do everything necessary to break the soul ties, you will be free. God has already paid the price, and your freedom is inevitable.

When you break those soul ties, repent and denounce them; take back what was yours that may have been stolen. God wants you fully restored and completely delivered at the same time.

First Things First

Surrender your life to Jesus and let Him rule over your soul. If there have been any covenants made by your words or actions, take some time to pray and begin to repent and denounce all the contacts you made.

Confess the soul ties out loud, accepting and covering them with the blood of Jesus Christ. It is washing you clean. Shut every door of fear with the Word of God and claim the promises of God. Fill your mind with the things of God, and throw away everything necessary that reminds you of that sin. *Keep your eyes upon the Lord and be intuitive* to the Holy Spirit; walk in the presence of God.

Good Soul Ties

As most soul ties are not beneficial for you, there are also good soul ties such as healthy relationships with friends. The body of Christ is connected when their souls are worshiping the one true God in one accord. They are connected when they are in agreement for righteousness and truth. That is a good spiritual connection. You can become tied to Christ by believing the written and spoken Word. In the book of Acts, 120 souls were connected in the same holy place, because all their hearts were in one accord. Anytime miracles, signs, or wonders occurred, it was when the body of Christ united, and it's still the same today.

Say this out loud:

"I renounce all covenants, pacts, promises, curses and every other work of darkness to which I have been exposed or made liable by my own actions or by the actions of others. By the act and decision of my own free will, Father, in the name of Jesus.

I ask you to go to the root and dig, cut, tear and loose me from every soul tie and from every form of bondage of my soul and body to the enemy.

Father, in the name of Jesus, I also, ask that you go to each of the above named, and at the root, dig, tear, cut and loose me from them.

I choose now to present my body to the Lord, as a living sacrifice as the Word instructs, and to walk in holiness as You, Lord Jesus, enable me to do so. "—paraphrased prayer by Nikki Jourdan.

As you follow all the above from your heart and don't give up, you will experience freedom and be on your way to a prosperous soul and the abundant life God has destined you to live.

Something to Ponder

Every connection on an intimate level you have ever had has tied you to their soul. You made a covenant with them and until the ties are severed forever, you will be forever joined with them, no matter what.

Action Item

Make it a point to go back to your past intimate relationships and break the ties (one by one) as God instructs you, until you are totally set free from all past covenant relationships. Take back what is yours as well: your victory, your freedom, your deliverance.

Words of Affirmation

"I am free from all negative soul ties and I declare every soul tie is destroyed in Jesus' mighty name."

Scripture

> "If the son therefore shall make you free, ye shall be free indeed."—John 8:36

Soul Tank

Root Cause #8—SoulWounds

The soul is the mind, the will and the emotions and can be wounded as easily, if not more so, than the body. A lot of your challenges and issues in life are due to unclosed soul wounds from your past. Wounds on your soul from ancestors could be dormant for generations. You may have been unable to hold a job, been rebellious, had needless, repeated negative reactions, allowed others to manipulate you, and had a fear of success; they could be a part of soul wounds that need to be healed, closed, and covered by the blood of Jesus.

Soul wounds are hindrances and blockages from moving into the destiny that God has for you. These blockages can become towering walls of protection so your soul cannot enjoy prosperity in your mind, will, and your emotions. Soul wounds are injuries that emotionally cripple and disable their victims. They can come from many sources and be inflicted at any point in your life. Some soul wounds are caused by a traumatic experience such as rape, molestation, abandonment, neglect, physical or verbal abuse, or by any negative or hurtful incidents. Soul wounds are bondages from past experiences that have never been closed and healed, and they can continue to linger and harm the fulfillment of prosperity in marriages, health, finances, and all relationships.

> "From the sole of your foot to the top of your head there is no soundness only wounds and welts and open sores, not cleansed or bandaged or soothed with oil. "—Isaiah 1:6

As with any trauma, the soul has experiences just as the body does. But while the body takes a wound visible to the eye, the soul takes a wound that remains invisible until it manifests physically. It is an emotional, mental, or willful bondage.

Covering Soul Wounds—The Blood

I was bathing my son one night, and he said, "Ouch, mommy that burns my foot. I have an open cut on my 'boo boo. '"Immediately I thought that when something of substance like salt or lemon touches an open wound, a burning or a pain takes place. A similar reaction can take place with an open soul wound. When a hurtful situation touches that wound, it burns, it stings, and it irritates the area on the soul.

If wounds are open, they are subject to the sensation of burning and stinging, which means, emotional and physical sickness and disease. Depression is rooted from a wound on the soul as well. Anything so deep-seated that you can't explain usually is from a wound on the soul. Repeated failed marriages and relationships can very well be issues of open gushing wounds. No longer think of wounds as a little "boo boo" or a minor cut.

Wounds are exposed areas that need a covering, like a bandage. In the flesh if you have a wound, you put a covering over it. You need to put a covering over a spiritual wound as well. The best and only covering for a soul wound is the blood of Jesus. If you cover the soul with the blood of Jesus, it is no longer exposed and subject to irritation. It will eventually, like any other wound, close up and be gone, be healed. You may have several wounds, and the blood of Jesus is powerful to cover every one of them until they are all closed up and gone forever. If any new wounds are revealed to you, immediately cover them without hesitation or thought by going to the blood of Jesus and the Word of God.

Other Soul Wounds

If your head is injured, there are signs you are to look for, such as swelling, hemorrhaging, and deformities. Consider that a head wound may not always be visible; it can be hidden. However, there can be internal bleeding, contusions, subdural hematomas, or other injuries, such as a concussion. How do you know when your mind is injured? You can't see into your mind. Your mind is the seat of thought and memory: the center of consciousness that generates thoughts, feelings, ideas, and perceptions, and stores knowledge and memories.

Many people are walking around with wounds to the mind resulting in negative feelings about a person, place, or thing, especially in memories. A person's memory is associated with the soul being toxic.

Sensory Memory

Sensory memory is the first type of memory that the brain uses to remember things. Sensory memory works when we see, hear, or even feel something. When you hear a song, it will take you back to a time or place either pleasant or unpleasant, depending on the association of the song and memory. Once this happens the brain decides to send this information to short-term or long-term memory.

Short-term Memory

The short term memory lasts up to a few minutes or only a few seconds. Once a memory reaches this area of the brain, it has been processed into a complex idea rather than an exact picture of what occurred. You may not have too many issues of toxicity here, since it is here and gone almost immediately. There is not a lot of storing in the short term memory; however, this is where the toxicity can begin. With one wrong thought, it can be transformed into your long term-memory bank.

For example, a married person may see an attractive person of the opposite sex. They can take the information in, and if they are smart, it's not stored; it is just a thought that doesn't take root. But if this person dwells and imagines being with that person, and if they take a mental picture of what they look like, smell like, or sound like, that is when it goes into a long term memory and gets rooted, causing issues in the soul.

Long-term Memory

This is the most dangerous and most deposited and stored area of a person's memory. This is where toxicity can take root and cause much damage to your soul. Long-term memory is where most of the action happens regarding the brain and remembering traumatic events in your life. They begin with encoding; much like a computer, you can record actual events and experiences into your long-term memory bank, such as colors, smells, and certain songs that are stored. You do have control in this area of your brain, and you do have a choice. The more you think about and dwell on the memories, the more they become stronger in your short-term memory.

They can then surface to where you are almost reliving the experience or event. Again, this is dangerous territory for the mind and can also have the tendency to lead to sin.

When Do Soul Wounds Begin?

Soul wounds can begin at birth or even in the womb. If a trauma takes place with your mother when she is pregnant with you, then you (the fetus) will actually be affected by this, and this is the beginning of the first soul wound. You had nothing to do with it.

For example, my mother lost my older brother from SIDS (sudden infant death syndrome) when she was carrying me in her womb. When I began to cleanse my soul, I realized the event of my mother's tragedy had actually affected me and scarred me in the womb, before I was even born.

When my mother was experiencing the trauma and loss of my brother, there was great sorrow and distress that I unknowingly received, and it became part of a wound to my soul. I have been delivered from this, but nevertheless, it was there at one time and caused many of the experiences and behaviors I had when I was growing up. My mother and I have always had a special bond, but it also was a bit overprotective at times. She was afraid to let me grow up and was fearful most of my childhood. She experienced a loss that no parent should ever have to go through. I internally suffered a lot of fearful times in my life as well, afraid to do many things on my own and always needing approval from my mother.

I am so grateful to God for showing me about the soul wounds I had and giving me knowledge about healing those wounds. God knows us intimately and knows what we need. He looks at our past wounds in our souls that are open and oozing. He died for our sins, taking on our wounds so we could be healed. As a follower of Christ, saved and delivered, you have authority over all the power of the enemy, and nothing shall by any means hurt you again(Luke 10:17, 19).

Closing up the wounds

- Forgive
- Repent
- Apply the blood of Jesus
- Let go of anger and bitterness
- Turn from wicked ways

It's really that easy.

Something to Ponder

Understand that Satan does not know you or anyone intimately; he only knows the weakness of the flesh. He can only recognize you by the open wounds that are obvious for him to see. Only God sees you through the cleansing of Jesus' blood intimately.

Action Items

Ask God to bring to your remembrance any past traumatic experience or loss, even since your childhood or maybe even in the womb. Then begin to work on closing those wounds with the Word of God and the blood of Jesus.

Words of Affirmation

"I repent for holding and carrying wounds to my soul and for wounding others. I am set free by the blood of Jesus and all wounds to my soul from the past are closed and sealed for good. "

Scripture

> "Moreover the light of the moon shall be as the light of the sun, and the light of the sun shall be sevenfold, as the light of seven days, in the day that the Lord bindeth up the breach of His people, and healeth the stroke of their wound. "—Isaiah 30:26

Part 2

Body Tank

Body Tank

Root Cause #9—Captivity or Freedom

Questions to ask yourself:

Am I living in captivity in my body? Is my body living in freedom? How toxic am I? Am I imprisoned by my own body's inability to eliminate? In order to effectively unlock the answers, you first must discover what a toxic body is, what it looks like, and how it becomes toxic in the first place.

Toxicity is the state or quality of being poisonous. If you are toxic from poison, what actually is considered "poison"? Poison can come from the air, food, and water, as well as different kinds of metals, leads, pesticides, hormones, nitrates, smog, cigarettes, drugs, and alcohol. Those and other contaminates can actually be in your body right now.

There are three major areas that your body receives and stores toxins. They are the skin, the colon (digestive system), and the lymphatic system. It is mandatory for your optimum health that you become aware of these following areas.

The Skin:

The human skin is a remarkable organ, the body's largest, but it is often taken for granted. Most people are content to let their skin be, not concerning themselves too much with the skin on any level unless it has some sort of condition such as rosacea, psoriasis, eczema, acne, a rash, or a wrinkle. These barely arouse any kind of attention. Once understood how the skin functions and the importance of the internal condition, on how it affects the external appearance, many may consider the quality and content of the skin care products they use.

If someone has dark circles, they automatically assume it is because of lack of sleep, which could be the case. What happens if the dark circles are caused from too much toxicity in the liver, due to lack of elimination and cleansing? Then how are those dark circles viewed?

The first line of defense in establishing health is the skin. It is visible to the human eye and usually will scream abnormalities in the body's internal systems. It's as simple as looking at the color of someone's skin. If it is with a healthy glow and a pinkish hue, that usually indicates wellness, and the body is operating as it should. If the skin is looking peaked or grayish and yellowing, that is an indication there could be something not allowing the body to perform as it should. This could be caused from a lack of proper nutrition, lack of elimination, or a vital organ that is being compromised. Immediate action should be taken.

Using natural skin care products can make more of a difference than most people realize. Everything you use or put on the skin is absorbed into your body. Take a look at antiperspirants.

The National Cancer Institute Study:

Aluminum-based compounds are used as the active ingredient in antiperspirants. These compounds form a temporary plug within the sweat duct that stops the flow of sweat to the skin's surface. Some research suggests that aluminum-based compounds, which are applied frequently and left on the skin near the breast, may be absorbed by the skin and cause estrogen-like (hormonal) effects. Because estrogen has the ability to promote the growth of breast cancer cells, some scientists have suggested that the aluminum-based compounds in antiperspirants may contribute to the development of breast cancer.

Consider These Facts:

- An adult's skin comprises between 15 and 20 percent of their total body weight.

- Each square centimeter has six million cells, 5,000 sensory points, 100 sweat glands, and 15 sebaceous glands.
- Skin is constantly being regenerated. A cell is born in the lower layer of the skin called the dermis, which is supplied with blood vessels and nerve ending. The cell migrates upward for about two weeks until it reaches the bottom portion of the epidermis, which is the outermost skin layer. The epidermis doesn't have blood vessels but does have nerve endings. The cell spends another two weeks in the epidermis, gradually flattening out and continuing to move toward the surface.
- Two to three billion skin cells are shed daily. The body expends this effort to replace skin every month because the skin constitutes the first line of defense against dehydration, infection, injuries, and temperature extremes. Skin cells can detoxify harmful substances with many of the same enzymatic processes the liver uses. The unbroken surface also prevents infectious organisms from penetrating into systemic circulation. As gatekeeper, the skin absorbs and uses nutrients applied topically. Because it cannot completely discriminate, the skin may absorb the synthetic chemicals often present in soaps, lotions, and other skin care products, which it has no use for and can be toxic or irritating. Skin is the first line of defense we visibly see when an issue arises with health or toxicity.

Most sickness and disease can be diagnosed just by the color of the skin or the overall appearance of the skin. It gives a visual snapshot into potential issues that may lie in the body.

The Colon:

The colon is made up of three main sections, housed within the abdomen. It is responsible for the final stages of the digestion process. It absorbs remaining water and electrolytes from indigestible food matter to accept and store food remains that were not digested in the small intestines and to eliminate waste. It is crucial to maintain a healthy digestive system, which is definitely connected to healthy weight loss, energy, clear young-looking skin, good bowel movements, and an overall vitality from organ to organ.

When the flora in the colon is not in proper balance with healthy bacteria, the end result may be constipation, gas, loose bowels, diverticulitis, and other disorders in the digestive tract. In many cases, when this occurs the body has too much bad bacteria and yeast, which is called Candida.

What happens when the colon does not function properly? The body's inability to eliminate properly is usually, but not always, a lack of proper nutrition, particularly a lack of fiber.

Constipation is the most common symptom of a sluggish colon. Hemorrhoids are enlarged veins, also caused by a lack of fiber in the diet and another symptom of a sluggish colon. Hemorrhoids are irritated by the difficulty in releasing waste materials. Colitis is a gastrointestinal disease that limits a person's lifelong diet. This illness is caused by an inflammation in the inner lining of the colon.

Halitosis, skin problems, and varicose veins are also caused by a poor functioning colon and indications the body needs to be detoxified. Since the colon rids the body of waste, it also cleanses the body. But most people live in a status quo condition and are used to living with constipation or diarrhea.

Beauty and the Beast—Fiber and the Colon

The beauty of fiber is that it nourishes the colon so much so that it can effectively eliminate all waste. The key to a healthy productive colon is food high in fiber. Fiber can absorb large amounts of water in the bowels, making stools softer and easier to pass. In almost all cases, increasing fiber in the diet will relieve constipation within hours or days.

Note: It is recommended that if you experience any of the above mentioned symptoms, you should seek medical counsel prior to going on any fiber specific diet or getting any other kind of treatment such as colonics. It is also advised to get regular screening for polyps as needed or recommended.

High Fiber Foods:

Apples with skin	1 medium	5. 0
Apricot	3 medium	1. 0
Apricots, dried	4 pieces	2. 9
Banana	1 medium	3. 9
Blueberries	1 cup	4. 2
Grains, Beans, Nuts & Seeds	Serving Size	Fiber (g)
Almonds	1 oz	4. 2
Black beans, cooked	1 cup	13. 9
Bran cereal	1 cup	19. 9
Bread, whole wheat	1 slice	2. 0
Brown rice, dry	1 cup	7. 9
Vegetables	Serving Size	Fiber (g)
Avocado (fruit)	1 medium	11. 8
Beets, cooked	1 cup	2. 8
Beet greens	1 cup	4. 2
Bok Choy, cooked	1 cup	2. 8
Broccoli, cooked	1 cup	4. 5
Brussels sprouts, cooked	1 cup	3. 6

Water:

Constipation and weight gain, lack of energy the remedy could be as simple as drinking more water. Everyone should be drinking at a minimum of 8–12 8-ounce glasses a day. Your body is 70 percent water and needs water to survive. If you are drinking less than that, you are dehydrated without knowing it, and you are automatically putting pressure on your vital organs.

The Lymphatic System:

The lymphatic system is the garbage disposal for your body. Your own body is a holding tank for fat, toxins, and disease. You are a walking waste dump. You take in nearly two to four pounds of waste per day, and most of that is made up of air, food, and non-filtered water. This does not include other chemicals, such as medications, alcohol, cigarettes, refined sugars, and other pollutants.

The lymphatic system is a storehouse. You actually store every illness that your body has ever had, even though you take antibiotics or other medications. Only the surface of the illness is being treated, enough so that the immune system can do its job properly, find and defend the body's antibodies. Eventually, the body functions again.

If only the surface of the illness is being treated, what happens to the illness or condition that is left over? The answer may surprise you: it goes dormant and is hidden in the lymphatic system. You keep getting the same illness over and over again because the illness is still in you but may not always be active. Poor nutrition, too many stored toxins, fast food, no exercise, too much stress, not enough sleep, and no preventive care are reasons for sickness.

Very seldom do people get a checkup from the neck down or just because they want to make sure they live a long healthy life. That, my friend, is called prevention. Most Americans would much rather take a pill for an illness than do what is actually needed, like exercise, detoxify, and eat right. It is not expensive to eat healthy and much less expensive than to eat bad food, like fast foods or processed boxed and canned goods. This type of care for your body costs money, time and discipline. If that were not the case the rate of obesity and diabetes would decline, instead of increase.

You can live into your late 90s and early 100s, but very few will actually make it. This all could be avoided and you could change your destiny with your health if you start to take a proactive approach and not be passive regarding the care of your lymphatic system and overall body's health.

According to the groundbreaking 2009 medical report *Death by Medicine,* by Drs. Gary Null, Carolyn Dean, Martin Feldman, Debora Rasio, and Dorothy Smith, 783,936 people in the United States die every year from conventional medicine mistakes or side effects. I don't know about you, but that is staggering to me, and I want no part of it. Do you?

If you are over 50 and take several medications, it is crucial that you do some sort of cleansing, either through diet or some other method. Cleansing with herbs or modalities that specialize in cleansing the internal systems is excellent. The average senior over 65 takes nine pills a day, and many of those pills are to offset other medications taken together.

The first place to begin is emptying the lymphatic system and making sure your digestion is properly functioning. It is very common in many to eliminate less than one time a week. They are told by their doctors it is normal, and that is just the way their body functions. That is not normal! You need more than one bowel movement per day; no exceptions, that is the rule. If you are not eliminating that frequently there is most likely a blockage in the lymphatic system that is not allowing the flow of waste through the digestive tract. It is time to take charge of your health and clean out those toxic tanks.

The lymphatic system assists to maintain fluid balance in the body, the main defense against disease, essential for weight loss, and enhanced immune system. The lymphatic system has several draining centers, or hubs, where the primary fluid collects and is stored. When working properly it assists in other areas of the body, such as the cardiovascular system where it increases blood flow and oxygen. It works in conjunction with the digestive tract. It can either enhance or lower immune system depending on the amount of drainage and release within the system. It has a direct effect on the elasticity in your skin, and it is the main cause of cellulite and weight issues, especially belly fat.

The lymphatic system is made up of a network of lymphatic vessels that carry lymph fluid, made up of waste, toxins and fat in the tissues and lymph nodes. The accompaniment of the lymphatic system is the spleen, which protects the body, clearing out worn red blood cells and other toxins and waste from the bloodstream to help fight off infection.

What happens to the infection once it is in remission? I say remission because it never really leaves; your lymphatic system holds on to the collective substance of the infection, and it remains dormant in the lymph system until it is reactivated by stress, or other factors that affect the immune system. If this process gets compromised and is not able to effectively release fluid and other wastes, then the end result will be build up in the body manifesting in the swelling of ankles and arms and retaining of water, called edema, or in some cases, lymphedema.

If you were to take an Italian sausage and tie up the casing and keep stuffing the sausage it would continue to swell and get blocked. That is exactly what your lymphatic system does when it is not cleansed regularly. Since your lymphatic system does not have a pump, it just continues to flow in an upward and downward movement towards the heart and never really goes anywhere.

Symptoms of a blocked lymphatic system are swelling, constipation, sluggish immune system, chronic, recurring sicknesses, cellulite, weight gain no matter the diet or exercise, acne, fatigue, varicose veins, sinusitis, digestive issues, and Candida—yeast problems.

When the lymphatic system is not being properly cleansed and released, it will become lax and sluggish, like a car that never gets an oil change. It will eventually not perform well: you will feel run down, your skin will have a yellowish/gray undertone, there will be a white coating on your tongue, you will have funguses and infections on a regular basis, and swelling in ankles and wrists, fingers, feet, legs and arm pits. Fatty tumors are also an end result to a blocked lymph system.

Releasing Centers/Hubs

Your lymphatic system has several releasing centers or hubs: the ankles, under the knees, groin, arm pits, breasts, gestational tubes, sinus, back of the head, abdomen, and kidneys. These specific areas are the most noticeable with fluid buildup, and become the most toxic areas in the lymphatic system. These areas prevent proper movement and flow of toxins to be purged that will diminish the health and optimal level of healing in the body. It detours the body's ability to perform efficiently.

A client came in with bloating and swelling in her ankles and unexpected weight gain while continuing her healthy lifestyle, with exercise four days a week, and eating healthy. She was desperate and frustrated that the weight was not coming off despite her efforts. She also mentioned she had unexplained fatigue, which made no sense since she was faithful to get her eight hours of REM sleep. We had determined it began when her father died, and it all seemed to go downhill. I knew instantly this was not only a physical trauma but an emotional one. She had undergone a traumatic stressful time for about a year as her dad's caregiver. Most caregivers are the sickest ones of all, because they are not focused on their own health but instead on the health of others, and they end up taking on more than they can handle; then their own health usually suffers. So we proceeded to talk, and she was dumfounded to find out about her lymphatic system and about it being blocked. We created movement in her lymphatic system and a series of sessions in order to take her to a maintenance level. Within weeks, she had lost all of her of weight, over 12 inches, acquired more energy, had restored elimination and felt better than ever.

Benefits of proper elimination and cleansing the lymphatic system

- More energy
- Inches and weight loss
- Better skin
- Less aches and pains
- Reduction or elimination of acid reflux
- Improved circulation
- Toning and firming

How a Healthy Lymph System Works

Lymph fluid drains into lymph capillaries, which are tiny vessels. The fluid is pushed along when a person breathes or the muscles contract. The lymph capillaries are very thin, and they have many tiny openings that allow gases, water, and nutrients to pass through to the surrounding cells, nourishing them and taking away waste products. When lymph fluid leaks through in this way it is called interstitial fluid.

Lymph vessels collect the interstitial fluid and then return it to the bloodstream by emptying it into large veins in the upper chest, near the neck.

Fighting Infection

Lymph fluid enters the lymph nodes, where macrophages fight off foreign bodies like bacteria, removing them from the bloodstream. After these substances have been filtered out, the lymph fluid leaves the lymph nodes and returns to the veins, where it reenters the bloodstream.

When a person has an infection, the germs collect in the lymph nodes. If the throat is infected, for example, the lymph nodes of the neck may swell. That's why doctors check for swollen lymph nodes (sometimes called swollen "glands"—but they're actually lymph nodes) in the neck when your throat is infected.

Problems of the Lymphatic System

Certain diseases can affect the lymph nodes, the spleen, or the collections of lymphoid tissue in certain areas of the body. The foods you eat make a difference in the lymphatic system. The average adult eats over 50 pounds of fried fatty foods a year Depending on your own diet, that amount may or may not be a lot to you. You may be wondering why foods matter so much. With your lymphatic system food not only effects elimination but also can add to cellulite issues. Since toxins and fat attract, the body can become more toxic because of the types of foods eaten. This can result in all kinds of external and internal issues of the body. That is why most Americans suffer with belly fat.

Weight Loss and the Lymphatic System

Diet, exercise, herbs, magic potions, and lotions, and nothing you do seem to be working. Frustration and desperation seem to be the only results for most. Sure, you can do a specific food program following some of the more popular ones being advertised today. However, if you stop eating those foods most of the time you will put more weight on, and it becomes a vicious cycle.

Instead, begin looking on the inside your body and not just what goes in your mouth. Since toxins and fat attract, when you take in toxins, because of every day foods, fat seems to just hold on, getting into your cells. It is like a guest that never leaves. Then one day you decide to clean house and toss everything out that doesn't belong, including the guest. It's similar in the lymphatic system. Most everything, including infections, goes dormant, always ready to recharge. If you truly cleanse your lymph system and maintain it, you will notice yourself becoming healthier, but you will also lose weight that will stay off. This is because you have opened up a system that has been closed up.

Are you ready for the change?

Something to Ponder

What state are you living in captivity or freedom? If you are living in captivity, then what are you going to do to change it? How will your life today improve if you focus on these areas on a regular basis and keep the body cleansed in for proper elimination and releasing of toxins?

Action Item

Take a moment every day to evaluate what you are doing to your body: are you drinking, smoking, and not getting enough movement?

Choose to eat one more gram of fiber, or start a cleanse or do something that will bring you one step closer to having freedom and not captivity in your body.

Words of Affirmation

"I will change what needs to change to have freedom in my body and overall health. "

Scripture

> "Who will transform our lowly body that it may be conformed to His glorious body, according to the working by which He is able even to subdue all things to Himself."—Philippians 3:21

Body Tank

Root Cause #10—Sugar

What's Eating You: Sugar, Sugar and More Sugar. . .

What is wrong with sugar? Sugar is a class of edible crystalline carbohydrates, mainly *sucrose*, *lactose*, and *fructose*, characterized by a sweet flavor. Sucrose in its refined form primarily comes from *sugar cane* and *sugar beet*. It and the other sugars are present in natural and refined forms in many foods, and the refined forms are also added to many food preparations. It is the refined part that is the problem in foods with sugar.

When it comes to choosing sugar, there is no doubt that unrefined raw sugar is the best choice. It contains minerals and nutrients that are stripped from refined white sugar and regular brown sugar. Raw sugar contains roughly eleven calories per teaspoon and has the same vitamin and mineral consistency that is found in the juice from the sugarcane plant. These minerals include phosphorus, calcium, iron, magnesium, and potassium. In addition, when sugar is refined and processed, there are many harmful ingredients that are added to it as a result. Some of these include phosphoric acid, sulfur dioxide, and formic acid. Unrefined raw sugar does not have any harmful chemicals added to it.

Sugar and Me—A Lovesick Story

"Hello my name is Nina Venturella, and I am a sugar addict. I crave sugar, I think about sugar. I can't wait to eat my meal so I can have my sugar, any sweets, cake, cookies, ice cream, but mainly chocolate. My real addiction is chocolate, but truly any sugar will suffice. "

The first step to recovery is to admit you have a problem! I have come to a painful realization that I can easily have a sugar addiction. I actually started getting back my symptoms of Candida that I have been totally cleared from for over ten years. The symptoms were coming back with vengeance.

The first thing I did once I realized sugar was addicting was to declare I was giving it up, and I also wrote it in my journal. I prayed for the desire to be taken away for sugar, I gave it to God, and I know that He will keep me accountable. When you have Candida, sugar is one of your worst enemies. It is no laughing matter. Sugar can be deadly and feeds disease, all cancers, and yeast, which cause sickness and eventually other diseases.

Once the choice is made, undoing any damage by sugar intake begins with detoxification. With every detox there is a withdrawal. I urge anyone who is going through a food addiction of any kind to begin today, even as you are reading this book. We will beat this thing to together! If your problem is overeating, binge eating, not eating at all, comfort eating, stress eating, you have the victory. With God all things are possible; just give it to Him. You are an over comer! You are never alone.

Step by Step—Ridding Your Addiction

- Acknowledge you have a problem
- Declare your victory
- Ask God to help you
- Surrender it fully to God
- Ask God to take away the desire for it
- Let God keep you accountable
- Make better healthier choices
- Do your best and take one day at a time
- Read the Word of God and declare His promises over yourself (out loud and daily)
- Be determined you have won
- Don't think about it just do it!
- Enjoy the victory; celebrate what God has done

It never works to attempt something on your own. God is your partner and will help you every step of the way. He will give you a complete victory; He has invested His entire life for you for all eternity! God is faithful, and you will prevail; you will have total and complete victory. "All things are possible with God."

Promises from the Word of God Re: Addictions:

"I am the head and not the tail."—Deuteronomy 28:13
"I am above only and not beneath."—Deuteronomy 28:13
"I am set free."—John 8:31–33
"I am victorious."—Revelation 21:7
"I am free from condemnation."—Romans 8:1
"I am strong in the Lord."–Ephesians 6:10
"I am more than a conqueror."—Romans 8:37

There are so many more promises; these are just a few to begin with. Read Psalm 91 and declare it over yourself daily. Receive God's protection and security for the just.

You Are What You Eat

You are what are you eating, and you are what "they" are eating. Don't just consider one level of the food chain. When you are considering what to eat, think about the deeper issue. If you eat bottom feeders, like shrimp or lobster, "they" ate garbage before you eat them. You eat what they eat. If you decide to have beef, what did that cow eat right before the slaughter? What about sushi and all raw fish? I know it tastes great, but at what expense, your health? Ask yourself that question the next time you order ahi tuna, or other raw fish.

The book of Genesis states, "Eat no unclean thing." God gave us all things pure and natural; nothing had pesticides, antibiotics, hormones, or pasteurization. It was all pure and without spot, just as Jesus Himself. Why do you think eight-year-old girls are developing faster and sooner than before? Over the years our foods have been tainted. It begins in the soil and what the animals graze on. I can't emphasize enough about the first level of our food source. The soil is not nutrient rich as it used to be back in the 1940s. You can no longer go to the store and expect to have the same nutrients or quality of food as you did "back in the day."That is why I encourage supplements and vitamins, because you can no longer get them in food.

Pesticides

Pesticides are substances or a mixture of substances intended for preventing, destroying, repelling, poisoning, or mitigating any pest. A pesticide may be a chemical substance, biological agent (such as a virus or bacterium), antimicrobial, disinfectant, or device used against any *pest*. Pests include *insects*, plant *pathogens*, weeds, *molluscs, birds, mammals, fish*, nematodes (*roundworms*), and *microbes* that destroy property, spread disease or are a *vector* for disease or cause a nuisance.

Almost everyone in the world is eating pesticides and is susceptible to disease just from the pesticides that are on the food. You probably were told as a child to eat your fruits and vegetables because if you did you would grow up big and strong. Maybe back in the '40s and '50s that was true. But today when you purchase fruits and vegetables, they need to be organic. Another precaution is to wash them really well before eating or cooking.

The FDA says there are not nearly enough pesticides to harm anyone. Believing them is your choice. Organic is the best alternative.

Organic anyone?

Organic foods are produced using methods that do not involve modern synthetic inputs such as synthetic pesticides and chemical fertilizers.

Raw Foods

Plant-based foods in their original, unheated (uncooked) state are considered raw and alive. Raw food may include fruits, vegetables, nuts, seeds, *sprouts*, grains and legumes in sprouted form, seaweed, *microalgae (such as spirulina and chlorella, etc.)*, and fresh juices. These live foods (living foods) contain a wide range of vital life force nutrients (vitamins, minerals, amino acids, oxygen) and live enzymes. Their nutritional properties are essential to the proper maintenance of human bodily functions.

Why Raw?

The benefits of going raw or vegan are boundless. Raw foods are easy to digest, and they provide the maximum amount of energy with minimal enzyme support. Studies have shown that living foods have healing properties that can alleviate many illnesses such as sluggishness, allergies, digestive disorders, weak immune system, high cholesterol, Candida, obesity and weight problems, and an alternative to chemo and radiation therapy for cancer patients.

The healthiest food today is uncooked, simply for the fact that the enzymes and the nutrients of the food have not been eliminated by the heating process while cooking. It is mandatory for a healthy digestive system as well. If a person takes ill with cancer or some other known immune challenge, eat raw fruits and vegetables, especially those high in vitamin a, c, and foliate; these vitamins and nutrients are the ones most eliminated when exposed to heat.

On the other hand, some other foods such as tomatoes are more beneficial to heat and produce more nutrients and benefits than when raw. Cooked tomatoes contain three to four times more lycopene than raw tomatoes. It also helps to eliminate any pesticides or other bacteria or harmful bugs that may be lingering around.

The choice is simply yours. When I am proactively trying to rid my body of something, I will for a few weeks eat raw only, and ease myself back to cooked foods. You must check with a nutritionist before you go on any extreme eating regimen. What's good for one person may not always be good for the other. We are all individual and have our own specific needs that must be met.

Preparing Raw Foods

Raw beans, nuts, and seeds contain enzyme inhibitors that are normally destroyed with cooking. The nutrients can be released by soaking them (germination) or sprouting them. Germination involves soaking in water for a specific amount of time. The recommended germination times vary from two hours (for cashews) up to one day (for beans). Rinse beans, nuts, legumes, or seeds and place in a glass container. Add room temperature purified water to cover and soak at room temperature overnight.

There are numerous benefits for going vegan or raw: beautiful skin and hair, cellulite reduction and healthy weight loss, and reduced risk of disease. The cellulite reduction is enough for me to start. What is going to motivate you to begin one of these programs?

Gluten or Gluten-free, That Is the Question

Gluten-free is eliminating all oats, wheat, rye, barley, or malt flavorings. Many people who have celiac disease must follow this diet in order to get relief of various symptoms such as digestive issues, lack of energy, bloating, and cramping. You will need to avoid fried foods because of the breading. A nice benefit in eliminating gluten is the loss of weight and lower cholesterol, which in turn will make you healthier.

Not only people who have these symptoms follow this program, but many others as well, since there are numerous amounts of health benefits. It has become extremely popular, even among the Hollywood crowd.

Do protein diets work?

The *American Journal of Clinical Nutrition* reported greater satisfaction, less hunger, and weight loss when fat was reduced to 20 percent of the total calories in their diets, protein was increased to 30 percent, and carbohydrates accounted for 50 percent. The study participants ate some 441 fewer calories a day when they followed this high-protein diet and regulated their own calorie intake.

The Atkins diet was the big craze in the '90s. Its popularity rose around the world, and many jumped on the band wagon for this protein-only diet. It worked for some and not for others. I believe the answer is simple. No two people are alike; what's good for one may not be good for the other.

Something to Ponder

"I am what I eat; I will carefully consider what I put in my body on a daily basis, and moderation is the key to my healthy body. "

Action Item

Go through your cupboards and pantries and look at all the labels. Toss out high fats and sugar-loaded foods. It is a great place to begin.

Words of Affirmation

"I am healthy, fit, and have a lot of energy. I eat only certain foods in moderation, and I am conscious of what I put in my body. "

Scripture

"Do not be wise in your own eyes; Fear the LORD and depart from evil. It will be health to your flesh, and strength to your bones. "—Proverbs 3:7

Body Tank

Root Cause #11—Yeast

The Silent Killer

In my past I struggled with Candida, an overgrowth of yeast and certain molds. In my research I discovered that most of the population today is suffering with this condition and are not being properly diagnosed. The reason is yeast is also mirrored with many other diseases and is the precursor to most diseases and most cancers.

Common Symptoms:

- Digestive issues
- Skin problems (infections, eczema, psoriasis, acne)
- Brain cloudiness (trouble concentrating)
- Chronic Fatigue
- Panic attacks (anxiety)

- Mood swings
- Obsessive compulsive disorder (OCD)
- depression
- Irritability
- Headaches
- Intense cravings(for sugars, sweets and breads)
- Itchy skin (hives)
- Sluggish immune system

Symptoms may vary from moderate to severe; some of the most common symptoms are chronic fatigue, acne, skin rashes, allergies, digestive issues, weight gain, and sluggish immune system.

Candida will progress and become more acute if not properly treated with the right diet and probiotics. It is important to note that yeast releases a special alcohol that depletes the body of crucial nutrients such as magnesium and potassium. Many clients have experienced shortness of breath and heart palpitations due to this alcohol. Unfortunately, this can also mimic heart disease, so many people are misdiagnosed.

Candida also depletes and doesn't allow the body to fully assimilate or absorb, mandatory nutrients that enhance the health in our body. Our food sources are not nutrient-rich enough, our soil is depleted, and too many additives are put in our foods. Processed foods, bleached, hydrogenated oils, antibiotics, and hormones, all play a vital part to the lack of nutrients in food. The only way to moderately get the nutrients you need is to buy totally organic or vegan foods. Too many bad bacteria (yeast) increase the probability of health declining rapidly in the body.

Host Environment for Candida

The prime environment that hosts yeast and molds is acidity. The talk around the water cooler is to drink alkaline water and enjoy all of its amazing benefits this water gives. I am a huge advocate of alkaline water. I also believe if you drink apple cider vinegar each day according to its recommended doses, it will do the same and create an alkaline environment in your body. Acid is what grows and houses bacteria and disease, and it also feeds cancer and provides a refuge for sugar to feed disease. An acidic environment promotes the growth of cancer, and infections become more active, which yeast feeds as well. Acid invades the colon and can cause colitis, Crohn's disease, irritable bowel syndrome, and other intestinal issues.

A normal pH should be 7. 0. If you take a proactive approach in keeping your body alkaline, the odds increase greatly for living a disease-free life. It will even be a challenge for the body to have any major health issues. Exploring the foods you eat, may provide the answers to what is causing an acid body and high pH level.

Citrus fruits are a good example. People say that lemons are too acidic; however, they are actually alkalizing because the minerals they leave behind after digestion help remove hydrogen ions, decreasing the acidity of the body. (The term "residue" or "ash" explains the effect of a food on the body. A food with an acid ash after digestion contributes hydrogen ions, making the body more acidic; a food with an alkaline ash after digestion removes hydrogen ions, making the body more alkaline.) Acid neutralizes acid.

Acid Forming Foods

Acid forming foods include asparagus, barley, beans (dried), beef, bread, buckwheat, butter, cashew nuts, cereals, cheese, chestnuts, chicken, chocolate, clams, cod liver oil, cottage cheese, cornmeal, cottonseed meal, crab, cream, eggs, farina, fish, flour, halibut, ham, hazelnuts, hominy, horseradish, Jell-O, lamb, lentils, lobster, mackerel, macaroni, maple syrup, margarine, mussels, mushrooms, oats, pasta, peanuts, peas, pecans, pistachios, pomegranate, pork, prunes, rice, rutabagas, rye, sauerkraut, salmon, scallops, smelt, smoked herring, sole, spaghetti, and especially *sugar*.

Alkalinity in the Blood

Alkaline forming foods include alfalfa (sprouts), almonds, apples (apple cider), apricots, artichokes, bananas, beets, blackberries, blueberries, broccoli, Brussels sprouts, burdock, cabbage, cantaloupe, carob, carrots, cauliflower, celery, chard, cherries, chives, coconut, cranberries, cucumbers, currants (fresh), dandelion greens, dates, dill, figs (dried), flaxseed, garlic, grapes, grapefruit, green beans (fresh), huckleberries, kelp, leeks, lemons, lettuce, lima beans (fresh), limes, mango, melons, mint, molasses, mustard greens, nectarines, okra, olives, olive oil, onions, oranges, papaya, parsley, parsnips, passion fruit, peaches, pears, pineapple, plums, pumpkin, radishes, raisins, raspberries, rhubarb, romaine lettuce, soybeans, spinach, squash, and strawberries.

Alkaline foods to assist in your journey of becoming healthier:

Extremely Alkaline and Alkaline Forming
Lemons, watermelon—great for colon health.

- Most all fruit listed (other than blueberries) are not allowed on a Candida program.
- Cantaloupe—does contain mold, (do not eat if on Candida program)
- Cayenne pepper—great for circulatory system

Celery, dates, figs, kelp, limes, mango, melons, papaya, parsley, seaweeds, seedless grapes (sweet), watercress.
Asparagus, grapes (sweet), kiwifruit, passion fruit, pears (sweet), pineapple, raisins, plums, and vegetable juices.

Moderately Alkaline

Apples (sweet), alfalfa sprouts, apricots, avocados, bananas (ripe), currants, dates, figs (fresh), garlic, grapefruit, grapes (less sweet), guavas, herbs (leafy green), lettuce (leafy green), nectarine, peaches (sweet), pears (less sweet), peas (fresh, sweet), pumpkin (sweet), sea salt on vegetables.

Apples (sour), beans (fresh, green), beets, bell peppers, broccoli, cabbage, carob, cauliflower, ginger (fresh), grapes (sour), lettuce (pale green), oranges, peaches (less sweet), peas (less sweet), potatoes (with skin), pumpkin (less sweet), raspberries, strawberries, squash, sweet corn (fresh), turnip, vinegar (apple cider).

Slightly Alkaline

Almonds, artichokes,Brussels sprouts, cherries, coconut (fresh), cucumbers, eggplant, honey (raw), leeks, mushrooms, okra, olives (ripe), onions, pickles (homemade), radishes, sea salt, spices, tomatoes (sweet), vinegar (sweet brown rice).

Chestnuts (dry, roasted), egg yolks (soft cooked), goat's milk and whey (raw), mayonnaise (homemade), olive oil, sesame seeds (whole), soy beans (dry), soy cheese, soy milk, sprouted grains, tofu, tomatoes (less sweet), and yeast (nutritional flakes).

Neutral

Butter (fresh, unsalted), cream (fresh, raw), cow's milk and whey (raw), margarine, oils (except olive), and yogurt (plain).

Moderately Acidic
Bananas (green), barley (rye), blueberries, bran, butter, cereals (unrefined), cheeses, crackers (unrefined rye, rice and wheat), cranberries, dried beans (mung, adzuki, pinto, kidney, garbanzo), dry coconut, egg whites, eggs whole (cooked hard), fructose, goat's milk (homogenized), honey (pasteurized), ketchup, maple syrup (unprocessed), milk (homogenized).

Molasses (unsulfured and organic), most nuts, mustard, oats (rye, organic), olives (pickled), pasta (whole grain), pastry (whole grain and honey), plums, popcorn (with salt and/or butter), potatoes, prunes, rice (basmati and brown), seeds (pumpkin, sunflower), soy sauce, and wheat bread (sprouted organic).

Extremely Acidic
Artificial sweeteners, beef, beer, breads, brown sugar, carbonated soft drinks, cereals (refined), chocolate, cigarettes and tobacco, coffee, cream of wheat (unrefined), custard (with white sugar), deer, drugs, fish, flour (white, wheat), fruit juices with sugar, jams, jellies, lamb.

Liquor, maple syrup (processed), molasses), pasta (white), pastries and cakes from white flour, pickles (commercial), pork, poultry, seafood, sugar (white), table salt (refined and iodized), tea (black), white bread, white vinegar (processed), whole wheat foods, wine, and yogurt (sweetened).

Potential Treatments

- Water filters

There are many water filtration systems on the market today. I suggest you research the costs and benefits you need and want. Water systems range from $100—$20,000. The price depends on the type of installation you choose, on the sink or installed into your plumbing.

- Apple cider vinegar

The daily recommendation is two teaspoons in eight ounces of filtered water, three times a day. For more severe conditions such as acid reflux, chronic cough, bronchitis, or sore throat, use one table-spoon of apple cider vinegar in eight ounces of water three times a day. For daily maintenance, weight loss, and pH balancing use two teaspoons of organic apple cider vinegar in 16 ounces of water per glass. This will keep your pH in a constant alkalized state by sipping this highly diluted dosage. If you drink a lot of water throughout the day, consider adding just a splash of apple cider vinegar to each glass or container each time you fill it.

Don't Feed the Yeast Beast

Sugar (all forms of sugars), fruits, and carbohydrates feed yeast. Candida Albicans is a form of yeast commonly found in the human body in the mouth and gastrointestinal tract. While the Candida Albicans yeast plays a vital role in the balance of the human system, so also does the good bacteria like Acidophilus, Lactobacillus, and Bifidus, which helps hold the yeast in balance and prevents yeast overgrowth. Yeast overgrowth can occur when the opportunistic Candida Albicans is allowed to grow unchecked and can cause symptoms ranging from headaches, fatigue, and joint aches to gastrointestinal problems and even depression.

The most common reason for Candida Albicans to grow unchecked and damage the body's good bacteria occurs from the use of birth control pills, antibiotics, chemotherapy, and a diet high in processed and refined foods.

Self-Test #1—Determine if you have Candida

1. How often do you consume dairy products?
2. How often do you consume breads?
3. How much fruit do you eat in a day?
4. How often do you eat sweets?
5. How often do you eat pastas and rice?

6. How many times do you drink, soda, coffee and caffeinated drinks?
7. How much alcohol do you drink?

If you answered "daily" to any of the above, you may be feeding yeast that is already in your body.

Self-Test #2—Body fluids

You heard it right—this is a spit test! You can try this simple test to find out. First thing in the morning on an empty stomach, with nothing in your mouth, fill a clear glass with room temperature purified or bottle water. Get a good amount of saliva from deep down and spit it into the glass of water. Check the water every 15 minutes or so for up to one hour.

If you have a potential problem, you will see strings (like legs) traveling down into the water from the saliva floating on the top; or "cloudy" saliva will sink to the bottom of the glass, or cloudy specks will seem to be suspended in the water.

If there are no strings and the saliva is still floating after at least one hour, you most likely have Candida under control.

Question	Yes	Score
1. Have you taken repeated or prolonged courses of antibacterial drugs?		4
2. Have you been bothered by recurrent vaginal, prostate, or urinary infections?		3
3. Do you feel "sick all over," yet the cause hasn't been found?		2
4. Are you bothered by hormone disturbances, including PMS, menstrual irregularities, sexual dysfunction, sugar craving, low body temperature, or fatigue?		2
5. Are you unusually sensitive to tobacco smoke, perfumes, colognes, and other chemical odors?		2
6. Are you bothered by memory or concentration problems? Do you sometimes feel "spaced out"?		2
7. Have you taken prolonged courses of prednisone or other steroids; or have you taken "the pill" for more than 3 years?		2
8. Do some foods disagree with you or trigger your symptoms?		1
9. Do you suffer with constipation, diarrhea, bloating, or abdominal pain?		1
10. Does your skin itch, tingle or burn; or is it unusually dry; or are you bothered by rashes?		1
Add up your score:		

Interpreting the Results

Women

A score of 9 or greater indicates that your health problems may be connected to a yeast overgrowth.

A score of 12 or higher suggests that they are almost certainly yeast cnnected.

Men

A score of 7 or greater indicates that your health problems may be connected to a yeast overgrowth.

A score of 10 or higher suggests that they are almost certainly yeast connected.

Foods to Eliminate

- Avoid eating sugar because it promotes the growth of yeast. The total carbohydrate intake per day is often limited. For example, during the initial two to three weeks on the diet, the carbohydrate intake may be restricted to less than 60 grams per day. Low-carbohydrate foods such as meat, chicken, turkey, shellfish, non-starchy vegetables, and certain nuts can be eaten.

- Avoid eating foods that contain any type of yeast. These include fermented foods such as cheese, tomato paste, mushrooms, and beer, bread made with Baker's yeast, Brewer's yeast, Engevita, Torula, and any other nutritional yeast. Other baked goods raised with yeast such as rolls, crackers, bagels, pastries and muffins should also be eliminated.

- Fruits contain natural sugars that support the growth of yeast. The following foods should be eliminated: frozen, canned, and dried fruit; all canned and frozen fruit juice; oranges and orange juice; melons, especially cantaloupe.

- Foods containing gluten are wheat, barley, and rye and include products made with these ingredients such as wheat bread, rye bread, and pasta.

- Vinegar is made with a yeast culture. Foods that contain vinegar include white vinegar, red wine vinegar, balsamic vinegar, mayonnaise, commercial salad dressing, ketchup, Worcestershire sauce, steak sauce, BBQ sauce, shrimp sauce, soy sauce, mustard, pickles, pickled vegetables, green olives, relishes, horseradish, mincemeat, and chili sauce.

- Mushrooms are fungi, which should be eliminated.

- Dairy Products: Candida is thought to impair the body's ability to digest fat, so dairy products may have to be restricted. How much dairy one consumes may also depend on individual reactions to cow's milk and cow's milk products such as cheese, yogurt, buttermilk, and butter. Temporarily eliminate the following dairy foods from the diet: cow's milk, including whole, skim, 2 percent, dry powdered milk, most cheeses. (cheese lower in lactose may be tolerated, such as Monterey Jack, sharp, white cheddar, Swiss, mozzarella, Colby, provolone, and dry curd cottage cheese.)

- Peanuts, peanut butter, and pistachios often have high mold contamination and should be eliminated.

- Alcoholic beverages provide sugar that feeds the yeast and stresses other organs such as the liver. Eliminate all forms of alcohol, including red wine, white wine, beer, whiskey, brandy, gin, scotch, any fermented liquor, vodka, rum, and all liqueurs.

- Coffee and black tea creates extra burdens for the body's stress-coping mechanisms. Regular coffee, instant coffee, decaffeinated coffee, and all types of black tea (including "fruit flavored" black tea) should be eliminated.

- Cider, root beer, and other fermented beverages should be eliminated. Healthy alternatives include water, vegetable broth, fresh vegetable juice, and herbal teas.

- Aged, moldy, and processed cheeses such as Roquefort and blue cheeses should be eliminated. Also eliminate processed cheese such as cheese slices, Velveeta, Cheese Whiz, cream cheese, cheese snacks, and Kraft dinners.

- Processed, dried, smoked, and pickled meats including smoked salmon, pickled herring, sausages, bacon, hot dogs, pastrami, bologna, sandwich meats, salami, corned beef, pickled tongue, and Kielbasa are processed and many contain unhealthy nitrates and nitrites, so they are not recommended for use at any time.

- Packaged, processed, and refined foods such as canned, bottled, packaged, boxed, and other processed foods usually contain yeast, refined sugar, refined flour, chemicals, and preservatives.

Allowable Foods for Candida

Vegetables:

All vegetables except mushrooms and all potatoes (one to two times a week; all skins should be scrubbed and then removed before cooking). Scrub all vegetables before use; peel or skin when possible.

Meats

Only consume beef in small amounts at a time. I recommend eating beef less than 3 times a month. You may eat lamb and crab, once a month, and salmon once a week. Turkey can be eaten as often as you like.

Dairy:

Butter Eggs Raw Cottage Cheese

Soy Milk Tofu

Condiments:

Apple cider vinegar (raw and unfiltered, refrigerated)

Fresh herbs (basil, parsley, etc.)

Sea salt, pepper, spices (without additives, MSG, etc.)

Homemade mayonnaise (recipe)

Beans & Legumes:

All (except fermented soy products, i. e., miso, tempeh); it's good to eliminate this group for the first month then eat only three times a week.

Fruits (one per day):

Apples *(Granny Smith-peeled)*Blueberries Coconut

Grapefruit Lemons & Limes

Oils:

Flaxseed, Sesame oil, Sunflower oil (just flavoring)

Olive oil (good for cooking)

Drinks:

Water-filtered & Mineral Herbal Teas (in moderation)

Nuts and Seeds:

Almonds Brazil Chestnuts

Hazelnuts Macadamia Pecans

Pumpkin Seeds Sunflower Seeds Walnut

Sesame Seeds

Sweeteners:

Stevia Xylitol

Grains:

Amaranth Barley*Brown rice

Buckwheat Millet Oats*

Pasta (whole grains that are not wheat) Quinoa

Rye*Wild rice Sourdough bread (recipe)

Pizza Crust (100 percent wheat and yeast free)
*If you are gluten intolerant eliminate barley, oats, rye, and spelt.

Miscellaneous:
Carob, unsweetened Salsa (fresh with no vinegar or sugar)

Adhere to the diet as closely as possible. Candida fungus grows on sugar, starch, and high carbohydrate foods and is fed by gluten-containing grains (wheat, oats, rye, and barley). Candida is also fed by the other yeast molds that are contained in many foods. Please read labels and check for ingredients that are on the avoid list.

Your cravings will slowly dissipate once the Candida begins leaving your body. After a month, slowly introduce foods back into your diet that are on the "Avoid" list. You will be able to tell which foods you can tolerate.

Treatments for Candida

Replace the good with the bad (bacteria) by becoming more alkaline and starving yeast with the right foods. You can learn to avoid the wrong foods and balance the bacteria in the body with proper probiotics.

Probiotics are good bacteria that replenish the body and create a balance in the intestinal system. There are different counts of probiotics and acidophilus; most need to be refrigerated.

Essential oils can help aid with replenishing good bacteria in the body, such as peppermint and caraway to ease digestive comfort. A hot cup of water with lemon will help add alkaline to your system and also help with the stimulation of your digestion. Ginger, fennel, and anise are used to normalize and stimulate digestion.

Detoxification Methods

In addition to balancing out the good and the bad bacteria, eliminate yeast by detoxifying the lymphatic system with my therapy X'Tract.

You can get colon hydrotherapy, which will aid in removing yeast that may be in the colon, which many times will come out in stools. If you look down after elimination you may see a stringy thick white substance, which very well could be yeast and in most cases is.

Another form of detoxification is to physically remove it with an ion technology cleanse, which effectively removes toxicity and yeast as well as parasitic properties from the body. I have seen results time and time again. I used this on myself and hundreds of people over the years, and many will testify that they did see and feel a tremendous difference. I had my own personal experiences with it as well. I invite you to take the challenge for yourself.

If you choose to do this, do your research. I have references on the machines that I recommend that work. They range from $100 and up; it depends on the type of machine and the use of it, and if it is for personal use only or commercial use. The price will reflect the use.

If you are proactive and do the above mentioned, I am sure you too will experience relief and be on your way to a healthier new you.

Something to Ponder

The yeast began to grow in me simply by taking a medication for acne. How many antibiotics or medications have you taken? How long have they been accumulating in your system? How many of these symptoms do you have, or ever have had in your life?

Action Item

Take inventory of all the foods you consume daily. Begin eliminating one at a time. When you're ready, do the full program for four weeks. Proceed to do the entire Candida foods list and menu.

Supplements

Use probiotics 50billion count or Bio K-Liquid drink (one a day), until you start to feel a soothing in your digestion. This allows the good bacteria to be replaced in the gut.

Suggestions: Ground flaxseed—for fiber and healthy elimination; coconut oil—for good fat for brain function and overall health; apple cider vinegar—to keep the body alkaline; stevia or agave nectar—good sweeteners; brown rice protein powder or egg white protein powder—for sufficient daily protein; BioK—source of probiotics.

Words of Affirmation:

"I am a healthy person. I have vitality; I have abundance in my soul. I have joy and victory in all I do. I do not crave sweets. I crave vegetables and good things for my body. I feel great. I will not give up! " (Repeat this daily, while looking in the mirror.)

Scripture to Memorize:

> "I can do all things through Christ who strengthens me."—Philippians 4:13

This is a much disciplined program; I did it for many years. You can do it because when we are weak He is strong.

Life after Candida

I can joyfully say there is life after Candida. You will be more focused, have more energy, and no longer have sickness due to too much yeast. It is all worth it. I promise!

Body Tank

Root Cause #12—Elimination

What Goes in Must Come Out!

Less is not more, especially in this case! Proper elimination is essential to one's health and well-being. I've had numerous cases where people came to my clinic with constipation. I saw people of all ages, but my youngest client was a five-year-old little boy, whose father came to me in a panic, ready to try anything for his little boy to move his bowels. The only thing I could do for him was tell him to drink more water and to increase his fiber intake and add fennel seed and psyllium husk. Carrot extract is also known to help move bowels. He had tried everything, including over-the-counter laxatives. Doctors couldn't help him except to suggest forcing bowel elimination with an enema, which is effective but temporary and very unpleasant.

When the body has this trouble eliminating, it usually means something more than occasional constipation. This little one had not had a bowel movement in over three weeks, and his father was concerned, as he should have been. More people need to take their lack of elimination more seriously. It is most times a sign or symptom of something else out of order in their body.

I had another case with a young girl who was 19 years old. Her mother found me in the yellow pages out of desperation when her daughter was extremely uncomfortable and bloated. After talking with them, I knew instantly it was her diet, how inactive she was, and her history with trauma both physically and emotionally. She had some trauma that resulted in a major surgery, and right after that the problem began. Her symptoms were bloating, weight gain, constipation, acne, and fatigue. This girl was beautiful, but she had never seen herself as that; she only saw the flaws. So I began my therapy of X'tract on her to see if we could give her some kind of relief. Within an hour she had produced a small bowel movement, and the bloating went down for a few days. We did a series of treatments, and to this day she and her mother are very good friends of mine, and we keep in touch. When they are in town I do X'tract on both her and her mother, which works well for them and relieves the issues they both had. The mother, by the way, had a slight case of edema in her ankles and lower legs; I was able to eliminate the swelling.

I had another case with a lady in her 60s. For years, in order to have a bowel movement, she had have a cup of coffee and a cigarette. She did this constantly for over 30 years and developed a trained habit for elimination. When she came to me, she said she no longer wanted to eliminate that way and wanted to quit her daily routine and go without the assistance of her aids. She had been trying to do so for some time, but her body was already trained with the coffee and cigarettes! We had a lot of retraining to do before she could eliminate on her own. I began correcting her environment, giving her probiotics and other herbs to assist in her elimination. We detoxified her and then performed many X'tract sessions on her to open up and retrain her body to correctly remove waste.

Many people are impatient and want results fast or overnight. The world lives in a fast food society: "I want it now and my way" that I like to call it soulish fast food method. It didn't happen overnight, and it's not going to change overnight; it will take time. I guarantee my clients would get results if they followed the program. The secret is consistency and a change in daily activities and mind sets.

Not having a bowel movement every day doesn't necessarily mean you're constipated. If you've had at least two of the following signs or symptoms for at least three of the past six months you most likely have constipation.

- Pass fewer than three stools a week
- Experience hard stools
- Strain excessively during bowel movements

- Experience a sense of rectal blockage
- Have a feeling of incomplete evacuation after having a bowel movement
- Need to use manual maneuvers to have a bowel movement, such as finger evacuation or manipulation of your lower abdomen

What is Constipation?

The most common of all intestinal issues is constipation; second to that are loose bowels. Constipation is not having the ability to move or soften stools and release bowels. Most women over the age of 60 have the most difficult time with bowel movements. Over four million Americans struggle with constipation or some type of release of bowels, according to the National Digestive Diseases Informational Clearinghouse. Suffering with mild constipation can often be helped by relaxation and waiting for bowels to do their thing, instead of forcing elimination or being frustrated. As food moves through the colon, the colon absorbs water from the food while it forms waste products, or stools. Muscle contractions in the colon then push the stool toward the rectum. By the time stools reach the rectum it is solid, because most of the water has been absorbed. That is why colon hydrotherapy is so effective: it gives the colon the hydration needed for proper elimination.

Common causes of constipation are lack of high fiber foods, not enough physical movement, side effects to certain medications, too much dairy (especially if you're lactic acid intolerant), too much yeast in the intestinal tract, as well as an acid environment in the body's system, gluten intolerance, and other intestinal issues such as irritable bowel syndrome. Clients have expressed concern with their elimination issues when they travel and when the overuse of laxatives or other substances to help in assistance with the colon no longer works for their aged bodies. The most common cause is not enough H_2O—water, water being one of the necessities of life besides air.

Foods for Healthy Elimination

Watermelon, broccoli, carrots, cabbage, kale, cauliflower, and artichokes, to name a few, are high in fiber. While high fiber foods are cleaning out your digestive system, some types of fiber bind with fats and toxins helps to cleanse your entire body. Many physical disorders, such as irregularity, constipation, and diverticulitis, can be avoided by getting enough high fiber foods in your diet.

All plant foods, such as fruits, vegetables, whole grains, seeds, and beans, have fiber. But all fiber is not the same. It can be divided into two categories with different effects on your body.

Soluble fiber is found in dried beans, peas, oats and oat bran, flaxseed, and phylum husks. It is also found in fruits such as oranges, apples, and vegetables like carrots. Soluble fiber binds with fatty acids in your stomach and prolongs digestion time. This helps to regulate blood sugar.

Insoluble fiber is found in whole wheat, wheat bran, vegetables such as cauliflower and green beans, and the skins of fruits and root vegetables. Insoluble fiber helps remove toxins from your colon and balance intestine acidity. It also helps move waste through your intestines and bowel.

HIGH FIBER FOODS LIST with TOTAL FIBER GRAMS (g)

Fresh & Dried Fruit	**Serving Size**	**Fiber (g)**
Apples with skin	1 medium	5. 0
Apricot	3 medium	1. 0
Apricots, dried	4 pieces	2. 9
Banana	1 medium	3. 9
Blueberries	1 cup	4. 2
Cantaloupe, cubes	1 cup	1. 3
Figs, dried	2 medium	3. 7
Grapefruit	1/2 medium	3. 1

Grains, Beans, Nuts & Seeds	**Serving Size**	**Fiber (g)**
Almonds	1 oz	4. 2
Black beans, cooked	1 cup	13. 9
Bran cereal	1 cup	19. 9
Bread, whole wheat	1 slice	2. 0
Brown rice, dry	1 cup	7. 9

Cashews	1 oz	1. 0
Flax seeds	3 Tbsp.	6. 9
Garbanzo beans, cooked	1 cup	5. 8
Kidney beans, cooked	1 cup	11. 6
Lentils, red cooked	1 cup	13. 6
Lima beans, cooked	1 cup	8. 6
Oats, rolled dry	1 cup	12. 0
Quinoa (seeds) dry	1/4 cup	6. 2
Quinoa, cooked	1 cup	8. 4
Pasta, whole wheat	1 cup	6. 3
Peanuts	1 oz	2. 3
Pistachio nuts	1 oz	3. 1
Pumpkin seeds	1/4 cup	4. 1
Soybeans, cooked	1 cup	8. 6
Sunflower seeds	1/4 cup	3. 0
Walnuts	1 oz	3. 1

Vegetables	**Serving Size**	**Fiber (g)**
Avocado (fruit)	1 medium	11. 8
Beets, cooked	1 cup	2. 8
Beet greens	1 cup	4. 2
Bok Choy, cooked	1 cup	2. 8
Broccoli, cooked	1 cup	4. 5
Brussels sprouts, cooked	1 cup	3. 6
Cabbage, cooked	1 cup	4. 2
Carrot	1 medium	2. 6
Carrot, cooked	1 cup	5. 2
Cauliflower, cooked	1 cup	3. 4

Cole slaw	1 cup	4. 0
Collard greens, cooked	1 cup	2. 6
Corn, sweet	1 cup	4. 6
Green beans	1 cup	4. 0
Celery	1 stalk	1. 1
Kale, cooked	1 cup	7. 2
Onions, raw	1 cup	2. 9
Peas, cooked	1 cup	8. 8
Peppers, sweet	1 cup	2. 6
Popcorn, air-popped	3 cups	3. 6
Potato, baked w/ skin	1 medium	4. 8
Spinach, cooked	1 cup	4. 3
Summer squash, cooked	1 cup	2. 5
Sweet potato, cooked	1 medium	4. 9
Swiss chard, cooked	1 cup	3. 7
Tomato	1 medium	1. 0
Winter squash, cooked	1 cup	6. 2
Zucchini, cooked	1 cup	2

Keep in mind many of these foods are not good for you if you have yeast or mold issues, so use wisdom and precaution when determining the foods that will benefit your nutritional needs and the direction and path you will take for process of elimination.

If you really want to feel good and lighter, but have more energy and a glowing complexion, then it is mandatory for you to eliminate daily and frequently. Use these food choices to help usher more fiber into your diet, and make sure it does not counteract any other issues you may be facing. As a rule your stools should look like letters, not pellets; they should be long and full of girth. If you do not have healthy bowel movements daily it is NOT considered normal. The body must rid itself of waste! If not you will become more and more toxic, which in itself has huge repercussions.

Many years ago I worked for the *New York Times* in Illinois. One day I had a very distraught man on the phone who had not received his morning paper. He very bluntly told me he cannot go to the bathroom and have his daily bowel movement without his paper! Maybe this technique is a little unorthodox, but it seemed to get the job done for him.

The bottom line here is it is not good to be constipated. If it continues longer than a few weeks, it may be more serious than just constipation, and further exploratory tests should be done. People need to take bowel movements seriously; theycan be a matter of health and vitality or sickness and disease, and in some cases, death. RELEASE, RELEASE, RELEASE!

If you carefully examine your diet and exercise—or in some cases, the lack of—all the toxins you take in on a daily basis, any alcohol, cigarettes, or medications, they all play a role in your colon and proper elimination. Over time, the colon can become impacted with layers of mucous, old fecal matter, and deadly toxins.

Considering the colon is an absorptive organ, toxins that are stored are transmitted to the blood stream via the millions of tiny blood vessels known as capillaries lining the bowel. These toxins settle in your tissues, contributing to a state of disease. This also has much to do with a blocked or sluggish lymphatic system.

Emotional Constipation

Emotions play a very serious part of healthy elimination. When the body is under heavy duress, it will cause an upset in the intestinal tract, which can either create constipation or loose bowels. Most all sicknesses, irregularity, and diseases on some level are affected by emotional issues or trauma that simply manifests itself physically.

Oftentimes when I did an X'tract on a client, there would be such a sense of release that they would start to cry, laugh, or both. They would ask me why this was happening. I simply told them that everything is connected to the soul, the mind, the will, and the emotions. When one area is released, it can bring different experiences about to the other areas.

Your soul can become constipated, and you can hinder or stop your growth in your walk with God, by holding on to waste. This can be caused by unforgiveness, anger, hatred, bitterness, and sorrow. This is the most important area for your body and mind to have health and vitality. If there is blockage in your soul, then there is a blockage in all other areas.

There May Be Parasites Inside

Parasites are organisms living on another; a plant or animal that lives on or in another, usually larger, host organism in a way that harms or is of no advantage to the host. There are several different types of parasites; each has their own symptoms and challenges accompanying them. There are over 100 different types of parasite worms that can live in human bodies.

Protozoa—There are more than 45,000 species of protozoa and many of these species are parasitic. More sickness, death, and suffering can occur with this parasite than any other. Intestinal protozoa are found often where water may be contaminated due to animal and human waste.

Helminthes—These include roundworms, tapeworms, flukes, and leeches. These are all wormlike creatures; the most well-known is trichinella, spiralis. It lives in animals in their muscle tissue. When humans eat infected, undercooked pork, they can end up with this nematode in their own intestinal tissue. The biggest of the parasitic roundworms is Ascaris lumbricoides, which grows up to a total length of fifteen inches in the small intestine.

Before entering humans, tapeworms use hosts such as fish, swine, or cattle that they may have entered through infected soil.

When the animal is killed for meat but cooked improperly and consumed by humans, it can develop into an adult that attaches to the intestinal lining of its new host.

Arachnids—Like mites, these can infest plants and animals. The chigger, a type of mite, leads to irritating rashes or bite wounds. Scabies can cause mange in some mammals. Female ticks attach themselves to animal hosts in order to suck blood. Ticks can carry diseases such as Rocky Mountain spotted fever, Colorado tick fever, and Lyme disease.

Parasites Causes

The first things to consider are food, pesticides, soil, and water; then mosquitoes and West Nile virus, a type of parasitic reaction to the nervous system, which simply shuts down when the virus invades the host. They rob the body of vital nutrients, so it becomes malnourished, struggling with keeping weight on or a lack of energy. If the host has a strong immune system, it can sometimes fight and defend against the parasite, but in many cases the parasite overtakes the immune system, and the host loses the battle, resulting in extreme sickness or in some cases, death. Most likely when a person travels out of the country, him or her most certainly will come back with some form of a parasite because of poor conditions in certain countries with water and food.

Parasite Prevention

Although this is not foolproof, it can definitely make a difference. Make a new habit of using three of your senses: smell, sight, and taste.

Smell your food. If it doesn't smell right or if there is a distinctive order, avoid it at all cost.

Look at the color of your food. If it looks old, the meat looks brown, if it is past its expiration date or nearing it, and it looks bad, avoid it at all cost.

Taste your food. If something doesn't taste quite right or is undercooked, then do not eat it.

Below are additional helpful hints for a proper elimination, so that you can look and feel better and live a more optimal life.

Wash your hands before cooking and before eating. You never know if what you just touched may be contaminated with roundworms or other parasites. Wash your hands after petting animals or after any contact with their saliva. That includes cats and dogs; it is known that cats are carriers of parasites.

Choose your vacation destinations carefully, and do not buy from unknown sources in other countries. Bring your own bottled water when possible. Do not eat anything suspicious or any unknown animal, vegetable, or fruit.

For extra precaution wash your vegetables before eating them raw.

Probiotics are live microorganisms thought to be beneficial to the host organism. When administered in adequate amounts, they can confer a health benefit on the host. Lactic acid bacteria (LAB) and bifido bacteria are the most common types of microbes used as probiotics. Probiotics are commonly consumed as part of fermented foods with specially added active live cultures, such as Greek yogurt, or Bio K as a dietary supplement, or Keifer.

Something to Ponder

Think about all the foods you eat on a daily basis. Think about how much you eliminate, or do not eliminate. Understand the methods you take to help elimination. Do you use any laxatives or other traditional ways? Take a full inventory of your bowel movements: how often you have them and what they look like.

Action Item

Eat more fiber. Check for parasites. Do not neglect your bowels if there is an issue. Check your stools daily until the situation is resolved. If not, seek other methods.

Words of affirmation

"I understand the importance of having healthy bowel movements and the responsibility I have to properly maintain my health. I declare my digestive system is daily functioning properly and I will continue to walk in wisdom and knowledge to maintain a healthy lifestyle. "

Scripture

> "My people are destroyed for a lack of knowledge."—Hosea 4:6

Root Cause #13—Trauma

Accidents Happen

When trauma takes place, it can be a root cause of sickness and disease and definitely part of the process of elimination. Trauma takes place when the body is under high levels of injury and the residual effects. It is a type of disconnect in communication in areas of the body. When the body is unbalanced with energy, Chinese herbalists call this *chi*. It is the life force of energy. You may have heard at times that one must balance out their chi. It is a fact that you do have energy in your body, and if there is an imbalance of that energy, it can very easily cause sickness and disease. This is a very important root cause that does need to be considered when using the process of elimination.

Within this chi are also pathways and meridians, which basically are trigger points in the body that cause upset in the systems. These meridians and pathways are not seen to the visible eye, although they do very much exist. It is similar to getting an EKG (and if you are over 50, you may have had this test). Electrocardiograms monitor your heart rhythms, which are just electrical currents, looking for any and all abnormalities. The chi is the same type of imbalance representing any abnormalities.

Again we are looking at blockages in the body that may cause a hiccup or in many cases, a severe, underlying issue in the body. This is another form of holding on to toxicity, only it is holding on to bad energy and not allowing for a natural flow. Unfortunately, we cannot see this imbalance until it is too late.

When chi flows freely through the meridians, the body is balanced and healthy, but if the energy becomes blocked, stagnated, or weakened, it can result in physical, mental, or emotional ill health. An imbalance in a person's body can result from inappropriate emotional responses such as excess anger, anxiety, and depression, and in more severe cases, suicide. Environmental factors such as cold, damp/humidity, wind, dryness, and heat can also cause imbalance, as well as factors such as wrong diet.

Meridians are the pathways of chi and blood flow through the body. Qi flows continuously from one meridian to another. Any break in the flow is an indication of imbalance. If a person's vitality or energy is recognizably diminished, it is an indication that the body's organs or tissues are functioning poorly; therefore, the chi flow is inadequate.

Twelve Major Meridians

The twelve major meridians correspond to specific human organs: kidneys, liver, spleen, heart, lungs, pericardium, bladder, gall bladder, stomach, small and large intestines, and the triple burner (body temperature regulator). Yin meridians flow upwards. Yang meridians flow downwards.

The Meridian Channels

Arm Tai Yin Lung Channel

If we look lung at the meridian, you will see it originates in the mid part of the body and it will move down, which communicates with the large intestine.

According to Traditional Chinese Medicine, the lung rules and regulates qi throughout the body and administers respiration (breathing). The lungs also move and adjust the water channels, so disorders of this meridian may be related to disharmony of lung fluid or "water" and respiratory disorders. Symptoms like chest discomfort with a fullness sensation, dyspnea (shortness of breath), cough, and wheezing indicate lung meridian disharmony. This disharmony can also lead to pain along the meridian position. For example, a person may feel pain in the shoulder and back or along the anterior border of the medial aspect of the arm. Specific symptoms include:

- Sensitivity, cough, asthma, blocked nose, headache, pains in the shoulders and back, pains in the arms
- Lateral chest pains, oppression, dyspnea, hemoptysis, sore throat and cold

Leg Tai Yin Spleen Meridian

The spleen meridian begins at the big toe and runs along the inside of the foot crossing the inner ankle. It then travels along the inner side of the lower leg and thigh. Once it enters the abdominal cavity, it internally connects with the spleen and continues upward to reach the Heart Meridian. Externally, the Spleen Meridian continues moving toward the chest and branches out to reach the throat and the root of the tongue. The peak time for the spleen is 9–11am.

Symptoms:

The spleen is responsible for the transformation and transportation of different substances and is the foundation of the after-birth existence. Spleen function is essential in maintaining the digestive power of the body and transforming food into chi and blood. If the spleen meridian does not function properly, chi cannot be efficiently transported to the spleen. As a result, symptoms like abdominal distention, loose stools, diarrhea, flatulence, and a heavy sensation in the body occur. In addition, symptoms such as pain at the root of the tongue, swelling of the inner side of the lower limb may also indicate disharmony of the spleen meridian. Specific symptoms include

- Stiffness and pain of the tongue, gastric pain, vomiting, jaundice, general weakness and feeling heavy
- Localized water retention particularly on the inner portion of the knees, stiffness or pains in the entire vertebral column

Arm Shao Yin Heart Meridian

The heart meridian starts from the heart and divides into three branches. One goes towards the small intestine. The second runs upwards along the throat towards the eyes. The third branch emerges under the arm and runs along the inner side of the forearm, elbow and upper arm. It then crosses the inner side of the wrist and palm and ends at the inside tip of the little finger, where it connects with the Small Intestine Meridian. The peak time for the Heart is from 11 am–1 pm.

Symptoms:

Disharmony of the heart meridian leads to pain at the heart position (precordial pain or pain at the sternum). In TCM, the heart rules the blood and the pulse. Without sufficient nourishment, an individual may feel thirsty and have a dry throat. Pain in the inner side of the forearm and heat in the palm may also indicate problems in this meridian. Specific symptoms include

- Dry throat, pain in the region of the heart of hypochondria, headaches with painful eyes, pains in the back, thirst, jaundice, hot palms

Leg Shao Yin Kidney Meridian

The kidney meridian starts from the inferior side of the small toe. Crossing the middle of the sole and the arch of the foot, it circles behind the inner ankle and travels along the innermost side of the lower leg and thigh, until it enters the body near the base of the backbone. After connecting with the kidney, it comes out at the pubic bone. Over the abdomen, it runs externally upwards until it reaches the upper part of the chest (the inner side of clavicle). A second branch emerges from the kidney and moves internally upwards and passes through the liver, diaphragm, lungs and throat, finally terminating at the root of the tongue. Another small branch divides from the lung to connect with the heart and the pericardium. The peak time for the kidneys is from 5–7pm.

Symptoms:

Disharmony of kidney meridian can manifest as wheezing or coughing because the kidneys "grasp the qi. " They also are the "mansion of fire and water," and the "residence of yin and yang. " If there is insufficient nourishment and warming of the kidney, symptoms like edema (swelling), constipation, and diarrhea can indicate an imbalance in this meridian. Pain in the groin and pharynx (throat), which are located along the meridian's pathway, also can indicate a problem with the kidney meridian. Specific symptoms include

- Lumbar back pain and at the base of the back, cold feet, haemoptysis, dyspnea, dry tongue, sore throat, lumbago, edema, constipation, diarrhea, motor paralysis and muscle atrophy of the lower limbs, hot plantar side of the foot and pain along the pathway of the meridian

Arm Jurying Pericardium Meridian

The pericardium is also called the "heart protector," and, for clinical purposes, is considered a yin organ paired with the yang organ san Jiao. In general theory, the pericardium is not distinguished from the heart. It is also the first line of defense against the heart from external pathogenic influences. The pericardium has a meridian named for it, which reflects the health of the organ. In terms of the five elements, these organs are both associated with the fire element. In treatment, it is often best to approach heart problems via the pericardium, rather than directly. The peak time for the pericardium is from 7pm to 9pm. Specific symptoms include

- Chest fullness, palpitation, irritability and agitation, spasm and contracture of the elbow and arm, hot palm and pain along the pathway of the meridian, stiff head and neck.

Leg Jue Yin Liver Meridian

The liver meridian starts from the top of the big toe and goes across the top of the foot. After crossing the inner ankle, it continues to go upwards along the inner side of the lower leg and the thigh, until it reaches the pubic region. It then circulates around the external genitalia and enters the lower abdomen. Afterwards, it goes up the abdomen and reaches the lower chest to connect with the liver and gall bladder. The meridian further travels upward along the throat and connects with the eyes. Finally it emerges from the forehead to reach the vertex of the head. One of its internal branches originates internally from the eye and moves downwards to the cheek where it curves around the inner surface of the lips. Another branch starts from the liver and passes through the diaphragm to reach the lung where it connects with the lung meridian and completes the cycle of the twelve meridians. The peak time for the liver is between 1am- 3am.

Symptoms:

Disharmony of the liver meridian leads to groin pain, chest fullness, urinary incontinence, difficulty urinating, swelling of the lower abdomen and hernias. Specific symptoms include

- Pulsatile headache, sneezing, blurred vision, tinnitus, lumbar back pain, vomiting, enuresis, urinary retention, hernia, pain in the lower abdomen

Arm Tai Yang Small Intestine Meridian

The small intestine meridian starts from the tip of the little finger and crosses the palm and wrist. It runs upwards along the posterior side of the forearm until it reaches the back of shoulder where it ends at the uppermost part of the back (the bottom of the neck). At this position, it first branches off and moves internally through the heart and stomach to reach the small intestine. The second branch travels externally across the neck and cheek until it reaches the outer corner of the eye and then enters the ear. A short branch in the cheek moves upward to the inner corner of the eye where it connects with the bladder meridian.

Symptoms:

Disharmony of the small intestine meridian presents mainly as symptoms along its pathway such as a swollen chin, stiff neck, sore throat, hearing problems, yellow eyes, and pain along the shoulder, upper arm, elbow and forearm. Specific symptoms include

- Pain in the inferior abdomen, reduce auditory acuity, stiffness of the back or the neck, easy tear formation, possible disorder of the sub-maxillary glands, pain or stiffness in the shoulders, frequent oral disease.

Leg Tai Yang Bladder Meridian

The bladder meridian starts at the inner side of the eye and goes across the forehead to reach the top of the head where it branches into the brain. The main channel then goes across the back of the head and divides into two branches. One branch crosses the center of the base of the neck and extends downwards parallel to the spine. Once in the lumbar region (bottom of the spine), it branches out to reach the bladder. The other branch crosses the back of the shoulder and runs downward on the outside, which is adjacent and parallel to the inner branch. It continues down until it reaches the buttocks where two branches run across the back of the thigh along different pathways that join at the back of the knee. The joint meridian then continues along the back of the lower leg, circles behind the outer ankle, runs along the outside of the foot and terminates on the lateral side of the tip of the small toe, where it connects with the kidney meridian.

Symptoms:

Disharmony of the bladder meridian can lead to problems of traditional Chinese medicine bladder dysfunction. It is often related to symptoms caused by external pernicious influences (outside influences that cause disease such as cold, wind, fire, dampness, dryness and summer heat). Because the Tai Yang Meridian is considered the most exterior, it is the first meridian to be invaded if there is any external attack. Therefore, its disharmony can cause symptoms such as difficult urination, incontinence, painful eyes, runny nose, nose bleeding and nasal congestion. Pain in the head, neck, back, groin and buttock areas indicate disharmony in the bladder meridian pathway. Specific symptoms include

- headache with neck stiffness, blocked nose and painful eyes, frequent tear formation, painful popliteal fossae, disorder of the calves
- Urinary retention, enuresis, pain along the pathway of the meridian

Arm Shao Yang Triple Heater Meridian

The triple heater meridian begins at the outer tip of the ring finger and goes along the back of the hand, wrist, forearm and upper arm, until it reaches the shoulder region where it branches off. One branch travels internally into the chest and passes through the pericardium and diaphragm uniting the upper, middle and lower heater (triple heater). The other branch runs externally up the side of the neck, circles the ear and face, and finally ends at the outer end of the eyebrow where it connects with the gall bladder meridian.

Symptoms:

Disharmony of the triple heater meridian leads to symptoms like abdominal distention, edema (swelling), urinary incontinence, difficulty urinating, loss of hearing, and ringing in the ears (tinnitus). Pain in the pharynx (throat), eyes, cheek, back of the ear, shoulder and the upper arm can occur as these structures are located along this meridian's pathway. Specific symptoms include

- Pains in the ears or behind the ears, swollen painful throat, stiffness or inflammation of the shoulders, enuresis, dysuria, reduced auditory acuity, ringing in the ears

Leg Shao Yang Gall Bladder Meridian

The gall bladder meridian starts from the outer corner of the eye and divides into two branches. One branch runs externally and weaves back and forth at the lateral side of the head. After curving behind the ear, it reaches the top of the shoulder and crosses the lateral side of rib cage and abdomen, until it ends up at the side of the hip. The other branch enters the cheek and runs internally downward, through the neck and chest to connect with the gall bladder. It continues moving downward and comes out in the lower abdomen, where it connects with the other branch at the hip. The hip branch then runs toward the lateral side of the thigh and lower leg. After crossing the ankle, it goes over the foot to reach to the tip of the fourth toe. Another small branch leaves the meridian and terminates at the big toe to connect with the liver meridian.

Symptoms:

In TCM, the gall bladder is closely related to the liver. Hence, the disharmony of the gall bladder meridian causes symptoms such as a bitter taste in the mouth, dizziness, headache, and pain at the outer angle of the eyelids. Pain along the meridian pathway such as in the axilla (armpit), chest, lower chest, buttocks and the lateral side of the lower limbs can also indicate a disorder of the Gall Bladder Meridian. Specific symptoms include

- Bitter taste in the mouth, dizziness, headache, infra-maxillary pain, pain at the external angle of the eye
- Pain in limbs, alternating hot and cold feelings, a fall in auditory acuity, ringing in the ears

Arm Yang Ming Large Intestine Meridian

The large intestine meridian starts from the tip of the index finger and runs between the thumb and the index finger. It then proceeds along the lateral side of the forearm and the anterior side of the upper arm, until it reaches the highest point of the shoulder. From there, it has two branches. One branch goes internally towards the lungs, diaphragm and large intestine. The other branch travels externally upwards where it passes the neck and cheek, and enters the lower teeth and gums. It then curves around the upper lip and crosses to the opposite side of the nose.

Symptoms:

Disharmony of the large intestine meridian can lead to symptoms of abdominal pain, intestinal cramping, diarrhea, constipation and dysentery. Since it passes through the oral cavity and the nose, symptoms like toothache, a runny nose, nosebleeds, and pain or heat along the meridian pathway can also indicate a disorder in this meridian. Specific symptoms include

- Abdominal pain, constipation, dysentery, pains in the throat, sore throat or pharyngitis, dental pains, red eyes, painful neck

Leg Yang Ming Stomach Meridian(Peak time: 7am—9am)

The stomach meridian starts from the end of the large intestine meridian at the side of the nose, and passes through the inner corner of the eye to emerge from the lower part of the eye. Going downward it enters the upper gum and curves around the lips and lower jaw. It then turns upwards, passing in front of the ear, until it reaches the corner of the forehead where it splits into an internal and external branch. The internal branch emerges from the lower jaw, running downward until it reaches its pertaining organ, the stomach. The external branch crosses the neck, chest, abdomen and groin where it goes further downward along the front of the thigh and the lower leg, until it reaches the top of the foot. Finally, it terminates at the lateral side of the tip of second toe. Another branch emerges from the top of the foot and ends at the big toe to connect with the spleen meridian.

Symptoms:

Stomach meridian disorders have symptoms of stomach ache, rapid digestion, hunger, nausea, vomiting, or thirst. Other symptoms that relate to disorders along the meridian pathway include abdominal distension, ascites (a fluid buildup in the abdomen), sore throat, nosebleeds, or pain in the chest or knee. Specific symptoms include

- edema of the limbs, cold at their extremities
- Pains in the legs, stomach pain, vomiting, facial paralysis, sore throat, epistaxis

From personal experience with many of my clients, this is the exact root cause of their sickness or disease. One minute they are fine; then a trauma takes place and disrupts the balance in the meridians. Disrupting the communication and connection in the meridians or pathways causes sickness or pain, and in many cases this can transpire years after the event. A delayed reaction can be because the body goes into such shock during and after a trauma, it takes that long for it to surface and recognize the damage done.

Why is it that a healthy young person, who hardly ever gets sick, has a lot of energy, never is in pain and always feels good, can all of sudden have sickness, pain, and fatigue after an accident of some kind? Think about it: doctors can't explain it, but it is real; they do have those symptoms that are there. The answer is a past trauma and an upset in the meridians and pathways.

How does all this information benefit someone? For example if you have surgical procedure and there are no complications whatsoever but all of sudden you're in pain, maybe your sciatica is acting up, or now you have swelling in your ankles or legs: can this all be related? Yes, it begins with a bruise, surgery, accident, or injury. Once a trauma of any degree happens, it is only a matter of time before one of the pathways gets interrupted and causes sickness or complications in the body.

Whenever there is a disconnection in the body and communication is disrupted, there will be issues—maybe not always severe—depending on the area of the injury or condition of the trauma.

It is important that we recognize the severity of the trauma as a root cause, since there are not too many people from birth that have not had a fall, bump, bruise, or even more of an injury. Many migraine headaches are the result of a prior injury that may have happened years ago, as many as 25 years later. The end result can be a sickness or disease that cannot be explained.

Something to Ponder

Every time your body has gone through any type of a trauma, even if is minor, there will be repercussions regardless of injury. The more time that goes by, the more the effects of trauma will take place due to pathways and meridians.

Action Item

Think back to every trauma you have ever had: where and when it took place, and look at the extent of the trauma. Then go to the description of meridians and pathways and you will see what the possible outcome could be.

Words of Affirmation

"I am balanced and all my pathways are free and clear for optimal health and healing in my body."

Scripture

> **"Do you know how the clouds are balanced, those wondrous works of Him who is perfect in knowledge?"—Job37:16**

Body Tank

Root Cause #14—Stress

Frazzled and Overwhelmed

Stress is the number one cause for sickness and terminal diseases. To determine if you currently are under stress and whether it is affecting your health, let's determine what stress is. Stress is designed to be a normal physical response to events that make you feel threatened or upset your balance in some way. When you sense danger, real or imagined, the body's defenses kick into high gear in a rapid, automatic process known as the "fight-or-flight" reaction, or the *stress response.*

The stress response is the body's way of protecting you. When working properly, it helps you stay focused, energetic, and alert. This is a reflex that can help save your life, or protect you from making a costly mistake.

The stress response also helps you to set your priorities in place, makes you more organized to be able to do daily activities and tasks.

Although too much of anything is never good, there is a danger being too over stress it takes a toll on your body's immune system, lowers your energy levels and can overload your body with toxins.

I have had a lot personal stress that resulted in my paying a visit to the local emergency room with a severe panic attack. It was probably one of the scariest episodes of my life, which I never want to repeat again. It was a few months after I opened my doors for my business. I slept fine through the night, but when I woke up my heart was beating unusually fast. All of a sudden I felt extreme heat and clamminess. I felt as though my arms and legs were giving out and, honestly, I thought that was the end for me. I instantly and abruptly called out to my husband who was in the same room and said "Call 911, I think I am dying!"

The doctor did many different tests and said my levels were perfect, my EKG was excellent, and they couldn't find anything physically wrong with me. It was nothing physical; the key was emotional. Not dying as I thought, instead I discovered I was having a panic attack. It manifested physically with symptoms of a heart attack, but it was an emotional attack. I was fine the next day! Now I don't get too serious about much of anything anymore. I stop and smell the roses and appreciate every day God gives me. As a matter of fact, I wake up every morning, thanking God for the day He has given me and my family. "This is the day the Lord hath made, I will rejoice and be extremely glad in it."

All have felt stress in some way at one time or another. Let's say right now you are in a great place, and all is well with you. Can you still be affected by stress? The answer is, "Yes." Stress is cumulative. Let's say you just got over a very intense, highly pressured situation. The residual stress from that particular situation can still be lingering, and it can cause havoc in your nervous system. It can cause reactions in your body, which in turn can cause sickness and in some cases disease. In my case it caused a trip to the local emergency room.

We define stress due to a prolonged response as chronic stress when the trigger is persistent or repetitive, not allowing the body to come back to normal by keeping the stress hormones at the higher level. The persistent stressors could be any one of the following:

- Workplace
- Relationships/home
- Financial

Stress is the body's reaction to any change that requires an adjustment or response. The body reacts to these changes with physical, mental, and emotional responses. Stress that continues without relief can lead to a condition called distress, which is a negative stress reaction. Distress can lead to physical symptoms including migraine headaches, upset stomach, elevated blood pressure, severe chest pain, and chronic sleeplessness.

Forty-three percent of all adults suffer adverse health effects from stress. Seventy-five to 90 percent of all doctor's office visits are for stress-related ailments and complaints. Stress can play a part in problems such as headaches, high blood pressure, heart problems, diabetes, skin conditions, asthma, arthritis, depression, and anxiety.

The Occupational Safety and Health Administration (OSHA) declared stress a hazard of the workplace. Stress costs American industry more than $300 billion annually. Just think if you were to lower your stress level and learn how to overcome the circumstances and problems of life. You would actually save a lot of money and time, and put energy toward a more productive cause like housing and feeding the homeless, for example. The statistics are staggering. The lifetime prevalence of an emotional disorder is more than 50 percent, often due to chronic, untreated stress reactions.

Cumulative stress on the body is called post-traumatic stress syndrome. When something tragic happens, such as a rape, accident, or a death of a loved one, it may not appear to affect you the way it may affect someone else. But your emotions may have been in a holding pattern, almost dormant. Then all of a sudden after the funeral and weeks go by, you may be doing something you do daily but this one time the reality of it all hits you. Your body goes into the reaction mode, and stress starts to take over your emotions, and in many cases, your physical body.

Effects of Stress / Physiology of Stress

When a person is exposed to a "dangerous" situation his body gets ready to face it. It needs more energy for that. The extra energy is received throughthe "fight or flight" response. The initial step is taken by the hypothalamus of the brain which secretes adrenocorticotrophic releasing hormone ARH. ARH stimulates the adjacent pituitary gland to secrete adrenocorticotrophic hormone (ACTH). This in turn stimulates the adrenal glands which are situated on the kidneys to secrete adrenaline and cortisol.

These two hormones work together to see that the body gets more energy by providing more oxygen and glucose. For these things to occur, the following adjustments are made:

- Diversion of the blood from less vital to more vital organs
- Increase in the heart rate to supply more blood quickly
- Increase in the blood pressure to supply blood efficiently
- Increase in the respiratory rate to get more oxygen from the atmosphere
- Breakdown of glycogen stores in liver and muscle to get more glucose

- Formation of more glucose from non carbohydrate substances

Foods Contributing to Stress

Foods that feed stress are anything with nitrates, like processed lunch meat, hot dogs, sausages, and high energy foods such as caffeine and chocolate. Chocolate does work on pheromones, so chocolate can sometimes do the reverse and ease your stress, depending on the person. Alcohol raises blood pressure but is another one that can either relax or increase stress again, depending on the individual. Dairy, such as milk and cheese, is one to avoid because pasteurization is not good for the body. And of course, sugar.

Foods that help reduce stress are most comfort foods, like an organic chicken pie, with fresh organic vegetables, turkey chili, pizza, and macaroni and cheese, which, although not healthy, relieves stress. Any foods you personally like that bring you to a happy place, or a good memory are considered foods that reduce stress (this is on the emotional level more than dietary).

Since most stress is pressure caused in the mind before the emotions are engaged, it is important that a person calm the mind down before reacting. Prayer and meditating on the Word of God and the promises that are rightfully yours are recommended.

Taking deep breaths in and exhaling all your issues out, to the point that you even over exaggerate your breathing techniques inhaling and exhaling. Exercise is a healthy escape and release from stress both on a physical and emotional level.

God's Way, Not the World's Way

The great question is, "What is God's way?" We already know billions upon billions is spent trying to cure or assist stress, which also encapsulates depression, suicide tendencies, fear, frustration, and captivity.

The only thing we can be sure of on this earth is that things, people, and places will always change, which in itself can be stressful. For example jobs, marriage, relationships, finances, health, safety . They can all change and be completely different in a moment's time. Wrong choices, wrong timing, bad economy, cheating spouse, bankruptcy, and sickness can change your world, but the only thing we can depend on to never change is God and His Word. He is the same today, yesterday, and forever.

If you put your faith in worldly things that will inevitably change, how can you ever know that everything is going to work out? You have nothing foundationally that is steady to stand on since everything you know can let you down through the process of life on earth and change. You cannot put your trust in the stock market because it are always changing, going up and down with no stability. You cannot put your trust in relationships as people have their choices. Even the weather is constantly changing! Yes, you can always count on God and His Word.

Relax Your Mind

It can help to write about things that are bothering you. Write or journal about stressful events and how they made you feel. This can help you find out what is causing your stress so you can find better ways to cope and find peace.

Let Your Feelings Out

Talk, laugh, cry, and express anger when you need to. Talking with friends, family, a counselor, or a member of the clergy about your feelings is a healthy way to relieve stress.

I spend time consulting with seniors and their wellness needs; a majority of my cliental is over 60. I often see some in their late 80s and 90s regressing and digressing in their activities or socialization. Many of these people have had very successful, busy lives and are no longer capable of doing those things. Many of them became depressed and very withdrawn. As I consult with them, I ask them what makes them happy. I often times encourage them to get out and try and enjoy life as much as possible.

Do something you enjoy often

- Hobby, such as gardening, bike riding, sewing, reading
- Creative activity, such as writing, crafts, art
- Playing with and caring for pets

Volunteer Work

As a volunteer, if you help people succeed in what they want or need, you will have more than what you need. You will always feel better when you stop looking at your own self, your own issues and turn your attention to someone else with a problem. We are blessed to be a blessing. In the book of Matthew, Jesus fed the multitude with a couple of loaves and fishes. Not only did He have enough to feed them but He multiplied with leftovers! Jesus gave the loaves and fishes to the disciples after He had received the blessing. He then allowed the disciples to bless and feed them themselves. We are blessed so we can bless others.

Blessing others is a sure fire way of reducing stress, because it takes you away from your own concerns and allows you to put the focus on someone else.

You may feel you're too busy to volunteer to help someone, but making time to do something you enjoy can help you relax. It may also help you accomplish things in other areas of your life.

When I have any type of pressure with stress or strife, I focus on anything but that subject or issue. I may take a walk or look at cookbooks, anything that helps me forget the problem. Maybe it is a hobby, a book, or a favorite movie, anything to divert your thoughts and focus. Confessing the promises of God and calling on the blood of Jesus gives me instant relief and an in dwelling of joy and peace.

If you want to tell if you are being led by God, look at the amount of joy and peace in your heart and life. I am not going to tell you this will all happen overnight, but I will tell you if you stick with it and continue to do some of these things to distract you, you will find you are no longer stressed, and there will be a calmness and peace in you.

There are herbal teas and remedies that also have been known to be very effective in reducing stress and anxiety. Herbal products and teas such as Kava Kava, Valerian, Dandelion, Chamomile, and Passion flower relaxes both the mind and the body. Chamomile, Lavender or Lemon essential oils can be put on the skin or infused. They work great as a tea also.

Something to Think About

Just because a person directs anger or some other disturbing emotion towards you does not mean it is about you. In most cases, it is their own junk they are dealing with, and you just happen to be in the line of fire. They are going to go off anyway; you are just there to intercept it. If that is one of your issues of stress in your life, just know you don't have to receive it. AND DON'T TAKE IT ANYMORE! Of course, you will want to smile and come back at them in love.

Action Item

Go out of your way every day to smile and show love to those who upset you or try to bring harm or discomfort to you. You know the old saying, "You reap what you sow."

Recommended Supplements

Herbal products such as kava kava, valerian, dandelion, chamomile, and passion flower relax both the mind and the body.

Essential oils such as lavender, lemon oil and chamomile are great as a tea, and can be put on the skin or infused.

Words of Affirmation

"I will refuse to let little things bother me or set me off into a tail spin. I will take things in stride and take it one day at a time. I will surrender this entire situation to God and lay it at His feet, and never take it back again. I will let go and let God. "

Scripture

"For God has not given you a spirit of fear, but of power and of love and of a sound mind."

—Timothy 1:7

Part 3

Spiritual Harvest

Spiritual Harvest

An Ocean or a Pool Analogy

It is here where you must make a decision to move forward in your journey with Christ in achieving the Trinity for Health, equality in the spirit, soul, and body.

Think of this analogy God gave me in my time of study with Him. The world is like a pool, and God's Kingdom is like an ocean. You have an opportunity to choose where you want to spend your time. I mean really spend your time, not just dip your toes in and out.

The question is ocean or pool; where do you dip your toes?

As a born-again new creation in Christ, I am constantly being reminded how much I need God and what my salvation really stands for. Anytime I have an issue or situation, I am forced to make a decision, either to go with God's will and God's wisdom or against Him with my will and what I think. Even though I choose God all the time, my emotions, my will, and my thoughts may occasionally show otherwise.

When there is a challenge in your life, your health, or your finances, where do you go to first? If you're sick, you go to a doctor or a hospital. If you are in debt, you go to a lender or some other source for funds. In either case you may decide to worry until you can't think straight.

Newsflash! Worry only adds to the problem and never solves it! If this is your protocol to a challenge—worry, confusion, anger, negative thoughts, rebellion or unforgiveness—then you are dipping your toe in the pool of the world, instead of the ocean of God.

You see, a pool is small, limited, has chemicals, and has to be continually cleaned, and cared for. The ocean is huge, vast, unlimited, and pure. God has filled it with salt and created the creatures of the sea to keep it clean.

If your protocol is to trust and rest in God, turning to Him, standing on the Word and not being moved, knowing your identity is in God and His Kingdom, then you can celebrate because are in the ocean.

Think back to a time when you were young and caught your first glimpse of anocean. You probably looked at it with amazement and excitement! You may have thought that it was something new and you couldn't wait to see what it was all about. That is how people are when they first get saved. It is new, and exciting, and they want to see what it is all about because they are so hungry for the truth. They literally can't stop talking about God and His goodness, and they are swimming around in His love.

They may begin to see how much they don't know, how really big the ocean is and they may get a bit overwhelmed by its difference, its size, and its magnitude. They begin to get drawn away from the ocean and find themselves back in the pool where they were more comfortable and familiar.

If they chose to submerge themselves in the ocean, they have to realize it takes real time and commitment; it is not an overnight transformation. Some people may think they don't have to put in the time, effort or make any sacrifices to develop their relationship with God, stay in the ocean, and not go back and dip their toes in the pool.

Unfortunately, the reality is that as time goes by and life happens they slowly begin to get out of the ocean and start to go back into the pool where they were most familiar. At first it is a small little "toe dip" and then they find it comfortable because it is what they have always known in the past. The pool becomes the norm for them. It is because they were born that way, and even though they have been saved, it is still easier and more comfortable to go back to the old nature and habits they are accustomed to.

Then that "toe dip" becomes a "foot dip" then a "leg dip" and before you know it you begin to splash around in the pool and are back to where you were before. It is so easy to just dip a toe in the pool and test the water, and if it feels good and make sense to your soul (mind, will and emotions); you decide to take the plunge full force back into the pool and leave the ocean.

I am talking about trust and faith in God and His Word with your entire health and life. You have to choose to stand on His Word, no matter what, because the Word of God is your final authority, always. God said it, and that settles it. It is done!

I have a quiz for you. For 30 days when you get a pain or feel sick, pay attention to where or who you turn to first. Is it God and His Word, or is it a person's opinion, a place, or a thing? Is it a chemical, a pill, or a drug? Do this for any and all issues that may arise calling for your immediate attention. Check to see who you turn to. Do you submerge yourself in the Ocean of God? Do you dip your toe in the pool and stay there, thinking that you know more than anyone? Maybe you'll find yourself going back and forth and dipping your toe in the pool and then back in the ocean. Are you all God, all the time, completely submerged in His Ocean no matter what? Dipping back and forth is exhausting. You simply need to pick the one you trust and stay there.

To be completely honest, I wish I could say that I never dip my toe in a pool. I definitely have been a "pool toe dipper," even in the smallest things. God is showing me how easy, fast and convenient it is to just go over to the other side and dip in the pool!

You may have said something that was not completely true. It probably was nothing terrible, but because you said what you said, you knew it was still a lie and a sin. It was a little white lie, and immediately as soon as those words came out of your mouth, dip, in went your toe in the pool. Because God is so faithful when you dip your toe in you begin to see the sin, and instantly you can choose to pull it out and submerge yourself back into the pure water of his ocean.

So the question remains, are you swimming in the pool or his ocean? When you dip your toe in, is it in the world, or is it in God's Kingdom? Where you dip your toe in the most is where you are spending the majority of your time (with your thoughts and with your energy).

So if you answered "pool," the metaphor for the world, that is where you have become the most comfortable and that is where you have placed your trust.

Then as time goes by the pool becomes even more comfortable, and you just go with the flow of things, not really anticipating anything at all. It may get you wet, temporarily refreshing you. Isn't that how most people react with their salvation while they still living in the world and the ways of the world?

As you get older, it should be easier for you to be wiser, learning from your experiences, understanding that you cannot live in both the ocean and the pool at the same time. How many times have you tried to do both and end up nearly drowning because there is no definite decision made?

You choose to jump in the pool where it's familiar; you know what you are doing, and you know what to expect. You become comfortable with the pool and the environment; you have been there and done that. You know there will be pleasure as you splash around in that pool. It becomes normal behavior to go swimming and play around in the pool of the world. You could think to yourself, "Everyone is doing it; it's no big deal."

The issue about the pool is that it doesn't last; it's just temporal. Everything in the ocean is eternal and never changes, but everything in the pool is just temporary. We constantly have to go to the pool to get wet and refreshed. The water eventually dries off, and we become hot, thirsty, and empty again.

The ocean, on the other hand, is a commitment. It takes more planning and preparing: you can't just jump in blindly, you don't always know what to expect, and the tide can take you for a ride without your permission. With God it is always a new journey. You simply need to trust Him, hold on tight, and let Him take you where He desires for you to go. If you trust in Him, you will never go wrong, never be thirsty, or ever need refreshing. Fresh streams of revelation will always be available.

What is the answer? How do you stay in the ocean and not dip your toe in the pool?

TCSR—Time, Commitment, Sacrifice, Relationship

Time—Spend your time wisely, thinking the right thoughts and saying the right words, being willing to be transformed by the Word of God.

Commitment—Commit your life to God and enjoy an intimate relationship with Him, studying the Word, renewing your mind and dying to yourself daily.

Sacrifice—Sacrifice the pleasures of the world, worldly ways and the things of the world that break your focus. Say “yes” to God and “no” to the world.

Relationship—Relationships needs nurturing, time, and trust. The most important and number one relationship you will ever have is with Jesus Christ. You can’t possibly have totally healthy relationships with your friends, family, or spouse without working at it and spending time with them. How could you expect to have a personal relationship with Christ without doing the same? You couldn’t. So go ahead and jump in the ocean where the water is pure, satisfying, faithful, unchangeable and truly great!

Spiritual Harvest

Abundant life

How does someone begin to live a healthy, whole, abundant life?

I had a Wellness Center for years and have had the privilege of working with many people. I have heard many stories and seen many versions of sick bodies. They all seem to have the same beginning and the same ending. “I just woke up this way,” “It came on suddenly,” “I have been like this for so many years,” or “You are my last resort.” (It was usually the result of some kind of trauma, physical or mental.)

When someone comes to me with an issue in their body, the first thing I recommend is to think back to when it all began to change, when it happened, or the exact time and moment the pain or sickness began. When you are a new patient and seeing a doctor for the first time you are usually given a stack of paper work, and asked about your history and your family’s history.

There are questions you need to ask yourself when trying to determine a timeline of sickness or injury:

When did I first notice the symptoms?
What emotional trauma did I go thru in my past?
Have I dealt with it?
Did I bury it deep down in my subconscious?
Am I still holding on to it, or did I release it?
Do I have unresolved issues?

That is the real issue, right there. Yes, you have a past and a history, and yes, there may have been some trauma associated with it, either physically or mentally. But the real issue is, are you still holding on to it, or have you let it go completely? If you have not let it go, then toxicity builds up, and you become blocked, and the waste cannot be released or eliminated. The toxins continue to be stored and eventually will become dormant until something brings it to the surface again. We serve an amazing God, who works all things for good, who even showed me how to turn around a toxic soul.

TOXIC:

T—Transformation of Body, Soul, Spirit

The spirit dictates what the soul should look like. The soul need to be transformed, because the natural mind clogs up our bodies. The journey of your soul needs to be changed and renewed. There is one God the Father, one Holy Spirit, and one Jesus Christ; they are three in one. I have often asked myself, "Why I am not seeing miracles, signs, and wonders like Jesus walked in every day?" He walked the earth as a human without spot, and pure and holy, and you are made in His image. I have come to a realization that it is our lack of faith, our wounded souls, our fleshly desires, our selfish motives, and unwillingness to love as Christ loved. It is also through His preparing us for our assignments, equipping us to do the work of the Kingdom, and humbling us when necessary; all done in His perfect timing.

> "With man this is impossible, but with God all things are possible."—Matthew 19:26

One of the most important ways you can be transformed is by choosing to follow in God's path and righteousness and saying, "Yes" to God no matter what; total submission to His ways, being renewed in the mind to the things of the Kingdom and not things of the world. You don't have any authority in God's timing, but you know He is never late, He is true to His Word, and if He said it, it will be done, according to His will.

To be completely transformed in all three areas, body, soul, and spirit, you must

1. Accept Christ as your Lord and Savior.
2. Spend time with Him and become intimate with Him.
3. Submit fully to His way and timing of things to come.
4. Allow Him to fully cleanse you and purify your body, soul and spirit.

You will be on your way to being completely transformed to a whole new you.

O—Overhaul Your Thoughts and Emotions

Your mind is a battlefield; the place where the seeds of good and bad thoughts are sown, or where they begin. In the garden Eve had to think it was a good idea to eat the forbidden fruit, and then the action followed. The battlefield started at the precise moment Eve ate of the tree of knowledge of good and evil; prior to that there was no thought of good or evil. Think about that. Up until Eve ate of that tree, there was not even a thought of anything but pure joy and goodness. It may sound like I'm picking on Eve, but she is the one who opened us up to the negative thoughts that we have been conditioned with since birth. She made a mistake that caused death, but Christ gave us another opportunity that caused life. One thought and foolish act changed our whole lives, by a thought that was transformed into an action that became a reality. That is exactly how it is today: it starts with a thought that we act upon, and then it becomes real.

So let's look at this in terms of your health. Can you actually think of yourself as being healthy or sick? If there is power in the tongue, then think about how much power and authority there is in the mind. Before you speak, you have to think of what to say first, and then your decision to take action comes. Depending on the course of the thought, whether good or bad, it will cause sin or blessings. If it is sin, or negative thoughts and actions, this will become rooted in your soul, which then causes soul wounds. I am convinced that sickness in your body is a mere manifestation of the mind, of thoughts and negative self-talk.

You have heard of mind over matter; this is mind over spirit. Your spirit has authority, not your flesh; your flesh is nothing but a covering, as a disguise to the nonbeliever of the glory light of God in our lives. As believers we are called to be the light of the earth. No one would be able to stand in the amazing glory of God, so He has us as His witnesses of His awesome light.

X—X-ray What Is Rooted in the Soul

Your soul is your mind, your will, and your emotions. Dissecting each of these, you will see the cause and effect of toxicity: negative thoughts, the tongue, gossip, anger, jealousy, greed, lust, perversion, immoral sexual behavior, using God's name in vain, fear, disobedience, unforgiveness, witchcraft, and unrighteousness.

As a sower, then, what are you sowing into your own life through your mind and your thoughts that are planted and taking root? What kind of fruit are you going to produce if the seeds you sow are toxic?

How about toxic fruit? This same fruit has the potential to go out and makes others toxic as well. You've heard the saying, "Misery loves company"? Well, it is even more so with toxicity. If that is the case, then it becomes a part of your own generational fruit, generational toxicity. Toxicity goes from generation to generation, because you can keep "sowing" poison into your own blood line, like pumping heroin into your veins; poison is poison. You may not dream of pumping drugs through your veins, but you send toxicity to your veins through your negative thoughts and hurt feelings.

> "And they shall receive the reward of unrighteousness, as they that count it pleasure to riot in the day time. Spots they are and blemishes, sporting themselves with their own deceptions while they feast with you. Having eyes full of

adultery and that cannot cease from sin, beguiling unstable souls, cursed children. "—Peter 2:13–14

Change your mind and you will change your life.

I—Ignite the Power and Authority of the Healing of God

The first thing you do when you are sick or in pain is to acknowledge that you don't feel well or that you are experiencing discomfort. Then you may seek out help from a doctor, or some form of professional who has been known to heal. Then you are examined, and a treatment or program for recovery is recommended. You may then go home if nothing is too serious and wait until it runs its course.

Scenario #2: you could be hospitalized, pumped with drugs, and surgery may be the recommendation.

Scenario #3: you could be told there is nothing that can be done, and the ailment is fatal and inoperable.

What happens when you hear those words in Scenario #3? Panic could set in, fear could attempt to take over your mind, and you have no choice but to wait for the ultimate day of death. If you are saved you have the comfort of knowing you will be in heaven with your Maker. If you're not born again, death is final and full of doom, and you are panic-stricken and unsure of what takes place next.

Let's look at the option that is successful for all sickness and disease, and all three scenarios, the healing power of the Spirit of God. If you are saved, then this is the obvious choice; if you are not saved, you have nothing to lose and everything to gain.

Remember back in the earlier chapters when I spoke of the Garden of Eden? This is our spiritual "makeover." You are born again, now not of sin or sickness but of blessings and wholeness. (John 13–17) The consuming fire of the Holy Spirit is waiting for you to access Him, have faith in the healing of your Father God, and step out into the destiny of wholeness and health that you are called to. It is the lack of authority and power exercised that is causing you to remain unhealthy in the body and the soul.

C—Cleanse

Purge, purify, refine, and apply all conditions of cleansing in the areas of the flesh and soul that must be clean and pure. With garbage disposals in the body and the soul, people hold on to junk, debris and baggage as if it were lifelines. People have been so comforted by what they know to be "true," that they dwell in the garbage and find a sort of solace within it. Why else do they hold on to bad things that consumed them at one time? Even dormant after an amount of time, deep down it is still there, waiting to surface once again. As long as you still hold on to that debris, you will never fully be clean.

Where does all the garbage go? In the body it goes into the lymphatic system, which ironically is the garbage disposal in the lymph system. It stores all the fat and toxins in the body and affects the entire digestive, immune, circulatory, and endocrinology system as well as weight issues. In the souls, it is stored in the mind, will, and emotions and memory banks.

The answer is simply this: clean house. God is known for cleaning out bad and starting over with the good. The blood of Jesus and Noah's ark are both examples of starting over; getting out the bad and putting in the good. God flooded the earth from sin and disobedience and started over new and clean. Why would anyone think that God would not continue to clean house in the things that matter to His children and His Kingdom?

Sodom and Gomorrah was a city turned into ashes, doing away with the filth and sin, receiving the reward of unrighteousness, spots, and blemishes. Most importantly Jesus died on the cross for our renewal and cleansing.

SOUL:

S—Salvation

The definition of salvation is the act of saving from harm, destruction, difficulty, or failure. Deliverance is another key word for true salvation; being delivered is the essence of who Jesus is and what He did on the cross. He took the world's sins in exchange for an abundant life and blessings. He purchased your sins, your sickness, and the curse of death in exchange for abundant life for all eternity.

It doesn't stop there, it just begins there! Most people stop at salvation and never get to the blessing and deliverance part of salvation. For instance, when I gave my life to Christ and said the sinner's prayer, I wasn't sure what to do next. I was told to get a Bible, go to church, find a good home Bible study, and have faith that God would do what His Word says. Even though that is all good, I didn't realize the awesome power and authority of Christ who now was dwelling within me. I never realized the power in the blood of Jesus and how I had direct access into the Kingdom of Heaven while here on earth. I did not receive the instructions on how to live the abundant life I desired to live, without lack in any area. I still was the same person on the outside, still living in the world, and still trying to figure it all out as a born-again Christian. I was basically clueless about God and life and how I should live it. Giving your life to Christ is only the beginning; salvation is the amazing beginning. There is a journey that begins; a journey into a supernatural, eternal life where you begin living heaven on earth.

O—Overhaul: A New Creature

Just what is a new creature? Throughout my Christian walk I kept hearing the words "new creature" and was confused and curious on what that really meant.

> "Therefore, if any man is in Christ, he is a new creation; the old has gone, the new has come."—2 Corinthians 5:17

You are no longer the fleshly person that has the same lusts and desires of the world; your flesh is dead, and your spirit is alive.

> "Therefore, if any man be in Christ" means to be united to Him by faith; or to be in Him as the branch is in the vine.

> "He cuts off every branch in me that bears no fruit, while every branch that does bear fruit he prunesso that it will be even more fruitful."—John 15:2

"Remain in me, as I also remain in you. No branch can bear fruit by itself; it must remain in the vine. Neither can you bear fruit unless you remain in me. "—John 15:4

"The new man, which after God is created in righteousness and true holiness."—Ephesians 4:24 (John 3:3, 5; Ephesians 2:10, 4:23; Col 3:10, 11)

As you are in Christ, so "God was in Christ" (2 Corinthians 5:19) hence He is the Mediator between you and God.

"Behold, I will create new heavens and a new earth. The former things will not be remembered, nor will they come to mind. "—Isaiah 65:17

So how does one respond to becoming a new creature? Do not blend in with the way the world does things. I will give you an example of new creature. I was at a party with my husband, and there was much alcohol, foul language, and sexual innuendos. I wanted to leave because my spirit was very uncomfortable, and there was a lack of peace in my soul. Deep down I knew I wasn't going to conform to the ways of the world and blend in with that party. I wanted to be the light in the darkness, and whether anyone at the party noticed or not, I will never know, but I knew my Heavenly Father saw. He sees all things; all darkness is revealed in His light. You can't fool God. You can't hide darkness; the light exposes it. He's always watching!

U—Uncover Truths about Toxicity

In my journey with health and wellness, I have learned a great deal about toxicity and our bodies, primarily in the lymphatic system and digestive tract. These are the most essential systems you have in determining your living an optimal, healthy life with established longevity. The cardiovascular system is associated with the lymphatic system and essential as well.

There are obvious methods of toxicity, such as foods, environment, Candida (mold, yeast), pesticides, lead, mercury, and asbestos. And then there are some other methods of toxicity that are not so obvious. These are negative thoughts, words, emotions, poor actions, anger, resentment, and jealousy, to name a few. In both cases you want to eliminate these and cleanse yourself from the inside out, spirit, soul, and body. Like most infections, it must surface before it can get eliminated. Once toxicity is established in the soul's lymphatic system and digestive tract, it becomes dormant until a trauma activates the infection or toxicity all over again. That is why many people keep having recurring illnesses or emotional issues. The toxins are still in you, but not visible anymore. So it's easy to just forget about it and move on with life, until another tragedy or trauma surfaces.

L—Lymphatic System or Garbage Disposal for the Body

Your own body is a holding tank for fat and toxins. You are a walking waste dump. You take in nearly two to four pounds of waste a day, and most of that is made up of the air, food, and water you consume, not including other chemicals, such as medications, alcohol, cigarettes, and sugars. What happens when you store all that garbage? I like to use this analogy: if you have a car, there is regular maintenance that must be done in order for the car to work and perform well. You put fuel in it to make it run. You change the plugs, and you even change the oil so that the car will perform and last a long time. So if you do all this maintenance to your car, what about the ultimate vehicle, the body? Why do you settle for just performing at a less than optimal level when you take better care of your car? You spend hours upon hours changing tires, doing maintenance checkups, oil changes, and lots of money to ensure the reliability of your vehicle to transport you from place to place. But many don't take care of themselves unless an issue arises! Very seldom do they do a checkup from the neck down. Preventative maintenance is to ensure you live a long healthy life.

Most people settle for living in the after effects, treating a symptom, which may be too late. This type of care for the body costs money, time, and much discipline to start eating healthy and working out. For most it can be too late and may end with some inoperable disease or being on medications for the rest of their lives. Is it worth it to care more for your car then your own body?

I am very passionate about this subject and get frustrated with the amount of treatment that is available to us, through medications, which can cause side effects. In many cases the side effects can be worse than the condition itself.

If you do have to take medications, and if your body does go through many traumas, then you need to begin cleansing! The first place to start is the lymphatic system to make sure your digestion is properly functioning. I can't tell you how common it is for many men and women to eliminate less than one time a week and they are told by their doctors it is normal and just the way their body functions. But I am here to tell you that is not normal! You need to have a bowel movement daily! It is recommended you have at least two to three healthy movements a day. If you are not eliminating that frequently, there is blockage in the lymphatic system, which is not allowing the flow of waste through the digestive tract.

Make the decision today to take charge of your health and put more care into your own body than you care for your automobile. This vehicle (your body) will get you farther with more miles than any car out there.

Appendix

Treatments That Cleanse

Electronic devices—One such electro-device that is very beneficial is a machine that delivers minute electrical impulses by a handheld device through the surface of the skin to the lymph nodes and lymphatic vessels. These electrical impulses help to stimulate the flow of lymph and break down toxins, making them easier to remove.

Rebounder—Basically a mini trampoline, a zero-impact exercise, rebounding that provides many benefits for you and your body.

This in my opinion is one of the best ways to exercise for toning, firming and ridding the body of toxins in the lymphatic system.

Dry Brushing

When you dry skin brushing, you actually help the stimulation of lymphatic fluid move, and helps to produce movement in the body. Although this is just the assistant to other methodologies for ridding the body of toxins, this will definitely enhance the progress with one of the mentioned methods used to release toxicity, such as X'Tract. You can look at this as homework in between sessions, or additional to any other methods you may choose to use.

BENEFITS OF DRY BRUSHING:

This process tightens skin, helps digestion, removes cellulite, and stimulates circulation.

Lymphatic Drainage

Lymphatic drainage is a holistic approach to promoting a healthy *lymphatic system* using light strokes and pressure. Lymphatic drainage is a type of therapy that is intended to help the body produce a free-flowing lymphatic system. In my opinion it is marginal at best in cleansing this system.

X'Tract

I have an amazing technique that will move the lymph fluid in the correct direction and bring it into the bladder, releasing all the hubs and resulting in the body's ability to effectively eliminate properly. This process is miraculous in the results it produced. I can't tell you exactly all of the benefits of this process only that it seemed to go to the weakest link in the body, whether it was swelling, eye issues, sinuses — it cleared them all. The one consistent result that all of my clients received was weight loss; it is the best way to lose weight and keep it off that I have ever seen. It is the miracle weight loss people desire. It works like this: the specific movement opens up the lymphatic system like never before. This is using only my hands, no surgeries, or tools or products, just using the hands God has gifted me with. I actually know how to train the lymphatic system to release properly and get it to a maintenance level so that the body will continue to perform effectively.

This is my own invention, and the Lord has given me permission to teach this and certify others with this technique, and it is being performed by certified TRC, Toxic Release Coach today. I will also add they too are getting the same results with their clients as I was. I believe it is because with this gift comes the anointing.

For more information

www.majesticwellnessacademy.com

THE MEANING OF X'Tract

X—Cancel

T—Toxic- involving something poisonous: relating to or containing a poison or toxin, causing serious harm or death (bacterial infections, candida) attraction of fat, feeding yeast with sugars. Toxic waste material can cause death or injury to living creatures. It spreads quite easily and can contaminate lakes and rivers—like living water—Holy Spirit. Toxins vary greatly in their severity, ranging from usually minor and acute to almost immediately deadly (Wikipedia definition) such as the power of the tongue, toxic voice, attitude, emotions, and physical body.

R—Release: free, resign, give up, unblock.

A—Accelerated: go faster: to move increasingly quickly, or cause something to do this. Progress faster: to happen or develop faster, or. The fluid is moving and directed at a rapid pace for proper elimination.

C—Cellular:(Bing dictionary) containing small parts or groups: relating to small parts or groups that make up a whole. Being completely renewed on a cellular level.

T—Transformation: Complete change, usually into something with an improved appearance or usefulness. Transforming the act or process of transforming somebody or something. Creating optimum performance in the entire body.

Young living oils

Grapefruit, Cyprus, release, energy,

Live five—probiotics

Power meal—brown rice protein powder

Seven Weeks to New You, Spirit, Soul and Body

Week 1

Stop, Look, and Listen

Stop what you are doing; it is obviously not working for you, or else you wouldn't be reading this book.

Look at yourself in the mirror, realizing you need to make some changes.

Listen to your own words and thoughts about yourself and others.

Acknowledge there are challenges you must face. Establish goals and desires for cleansing each of the tanks.

Begin the process of elimination.

Week 2

You have acknowledged you have certain challenges and have become toxic in certain areas. It is important that you work on one tank at a time.

Do all the tasks at the end of each chapter. This is a how-to book so at the end of the seven weeks you will be a different person. You will never be the same again. Journal all your findings and write down all your goals.

Read the scriptures that are recommended at the end of this book and ask the Holy Spirit to give you a level of understanding and revelation on how this applies directly to you.

Week 3

This is the week when you will go over all the affirmations and promises that God has given you about your health and well-being.

You will begin to reestablish your goals and desires with your cleanse. If you need to change anything in your diet, this is also the week to focus on that.

Week 4

You're more than halfway there! This is the week you renounce all the generational curses and break all soul ties. You will focus every day on breaking free and cleansing this tank.

Week 5

You may possibly feel some of the side effects of the tanks being cleansed. This week keep doing what you are doing and don't give up! This is a crucial week. You're almost there! Focus on Luke 10:17, 19 and your daily affirmation should be "No weapon formed against me shall prosper." I also recommend you start wearing your armor found in Ephesians 6:10–18. You are so close to your breakthrough; keep up the good work!

Week 6

You are ready to start focusing on cleansing your lymphatic system and colon. Focus on the body tank this week. Make appointments for your therapies, take a trip to your health food store and pick up a "colon cleanse kit." This week is dedicated to making sure your physical tank is completely cleansed.

Week 7

Congratulations! You made it. By this time you have cleansed all three tanks, you have endured the detoxification process, and you are on your way to a healthy you; body, soul and spirit.

Use this book over and over again, going back to any of the weeks when necessary, for a tune up. If used properly, this book will benefit you all the days of your life.

Seven Weeks, the Sign of Complete Perfection

When man began to analyze and combine numbers, he developed other interesting symbols. He took the perfect world number added to it the perfect divine number three, and got seven; the most sacred number to the Hebrews. It was earth crowned with heaven: the four-square earth plus the divine completeness of God. The number seven expresses completeness through the union of earth and heaven. This number is used more than all other numbers in the word of God, except the number one.

In the Book of Revelation the number seven is used throughout. There are seven churches, seven spirits, seven stars, seven seals, seven trumpets, seven vials, seven personages, seven dooms, and seven new things. The number seven symbolizes spiritual perfection. All of life revolves around this number. Seven is used over 700 times in the Bible. It is used 54 times in the Book of Revelation.

The whole Word of God is founded upon the number seven. It stands for the seventh day of the creation week, and speaks of the millennial rest day. It denotes completeness or perfection.

Spiritual Food-The food that heals every disease

Spiritual food is your bread of life. It is the holy written Word of God; it is your substance for all your wants and needs. Spiritual food fills you up, both in natural and supernatural ways. I have noticed when the glory of God comes and His presence is on me, that I am satisfied completely. I don't need anything but Him; I am not hungry, thirsty, tired, or in pain; absolutely wanting nothing.

Normally my flesh needs something to eat at least every three hours; I trained it that way. I eat three square meals and two or three snacks a day. I drink at least ten glasses of water a day, a necessity for my body to function well. Food and water are essential for survival. If you are in touch with your body, you know when you must eat and drink water, and if not, it will not function and feel right. Your urine will represent lack of fluid, and your energy will represent the lack of food. If you are hypoglycemic, it means your sugar drops if you do not get what you need in terms of food prior to that point of feeling shaky or moody.

We have God's Word and His presence to give the spirit what it needs through the spiritual feeding of the presence of the Holy Spirit. He quenches your thirst; He feeds your spirit with His Word, "Not by bread alone, but by every Word that proceeds out the mouth of the Lord." It is true with natural food and thirst, and it is true with the healing in all of the flesh, all through the Spirit. Your body is transformed by the Spirit when you are in His presence. There is no time clock or even a concept of time; a thousand years is like a day in heaven. So it makes sense for total restoration to take place in the body and in people's lives while in His presence.

Living in His presence is an everyday continual state of being with the Father; daily visits into His throne room, His voice speaking to His inherited children of the Kingdom. Total and complete transformation takes place in the Kingdom, and it's there that the Kingdom is established in you. If you abide in the Kingdom, established in the presence of the Holy Spirit, feeding on His Word (which cannot return void), then your spiritual food is Christ Himself. He is all sufficient for your every need. He is the only satisfying food you ever really need.

All healing takes place when His presence is in you and on you, for you, and for others. It is the normal response for the body to be healed, because it already has all it needs to live the healthy whole life you are designed for. Your salvation is all inclusive, wrapped in God's love through the blood of the Lamb. The blood of the Lamb was shed for you, for your salvation, healing, deliverance, redemption, restoration, and provision.

There has been an exchange that the blood has given you. Jesus, the Son of God, who died on the cross for your sins, not only died for you to have eternal life, but also so that you can have all the things associated with the blood. The blood is what brings you into your rightful inheritance as children of the family of God.

> "My people are destroyed because of lack of knowledge."—Hosea 4:6

Understanding what the blood has done for you and what the cross represents for you is crucial for living the abundant, toxic-free life Christ purchased for you.

Many know of salvation, the crucifixion, and the resurrection, but for many it stops there. They try to live a good life, treat people well, and expect to go to heaven. For many that is their entire walk and relationship with God; He is acknowledged, celebrated on special occasions and holidays; they go to church on Sundays and give offerings occasionally. That's not the abundant life in Christ.

In order to really grasp what the cross accomplished for you and His blood did for you, you need to seek Him. Your life needs to be all about Him, spending time with Him. He not only desires an intimate relationship with you, He created you for Himself. God desires His children to overcome the world.

"For whosoever is born of God overcomes the world; and this is the victory that overcomes the world even our faith."—1 John 5: 4

Victory is God's plan for your life. Victory is God's plan for your health. What does victory look like in your body? Are sickness and pain the norm; are they accepted and the status quo now? Is a watered-down version of healthy all that is available?

Having my Wellness Center and seeing hundreds of clients a month, I heard many stories and have seen many versions of sick bodies. They all seemed to have the same beginning and same ending, "I just woke up this way," "It came on suddenly," "I have been like this for so many years," "You are my last resort," or "It all seemed to start after this happened to me." They all began with an incident that impacted them or a trauma (physical or emotional).

If you go to a doctor, they will give you a form and ask about your family history. "When did this problem begin?" That is the first question you need to ask yourself. When did you first notice the symptoms? What emotional trauma did you go through in your past? Have you dealt with it, or did you bury it deep down in your subconscious? Are you holding on to it or did you release it? That is the real issue. You have a past, and you have a history. There may have been some trauma associated with your life, either physically or mentally. But the real question is, do you still hold on to it, or have you let it go?

pg. 72. Explain the desire for more, and how do you know we were born w/ it?

Can you break soul ties w/ anybody? Let's talk

Don't understand fully all the accounts but I want to break soul ties w/ all the men of my past

CPSIA information can be obtained at www.ICGtesting.com
Printed in the USA
BVOW04s1301081014

369972BV00001B/148/P